Contemporary Diagnosis and Management of Fungal Infections®

Jack D. Sobel, MD
Chief, Division of Infectious Diseases
and Professor of Internal Medicine,
Detroit Medical Center
Wayne State University School of Medicine
Detroit, Michigan

José A. Vazquez, MD
Senior Staff, Division of Infectious Diseases
Henry Ford Hospital
Professor of Medicine,
Wayne State University School of Medicine
Detroit, Michigan

Third Edition

Published by Handbooks in Health Care Co.,
Newtown, Pennsylvania, USA

This book has been prepared and is presented as a service to the medical community. The information provided reflects the knowledge, experience, and personal opinions of the authors, Jack D. Sobel, MD, Professor of Medicine, Division of Infectious Diseases, Wayne State University School of Medicine, Detroit Medical Center, Division of Infectious Diseases, Detroit, Michigan, and José A. Vazquez, MD, Senior Staff, Division of Infectious Diseases, Henry Ford Hospital, Professor of Medicine, Wayne State University School of Medicine, Division of Infectious Diseases, Detroit.

This book is not intended to replace or to be used as a substitute for the complete prescribing information prepared by each manufacturer for each drug. Because of possible variations in drug indications, in dosage information, in newly described toxicities, in drug/drug interactions, and in other items of importance, reference to such complete prescribing information is definitely recommended before any of the drugs discussed are used or prescribed.

International Standard Book Number: 978-1-935103-26-4

Library of Congress Catalog Card Number: 2009927453

Table of Contents

Chapter 1

Introduction

Fungi are ubiquitous in plants, mammals, and insects. Consequently, humans are continually exposed to numerous genera of fungi through a variety of routes. Depending on the interaction between human host defense mechanisms and fungal virulence factors, colonization may progress to either local disease or, occasionally, to disseminated infection.

Advances in medical technology, chemotherapy, cancer therapy, and organ transplantation have substantially reduced the morbidity and mortality of life-threatening fungal disease. Along with these benefits, however, has emerged a variety of opportunistic infections frequently caused by relatively avirulent organisms. Critically ill, immunocompromised patients are the prime targets for these opportunistic fungal infections, primarily due to *Candida* and *Aspergillus* species. Recent epidemiologic studies suggest that the mortality rate from invasive fungal infections is increasing. Most physicians are confronted daily with a patient who has a positive fungal culture obtained from one or more anatomical sites.

Clinical and autopsy studies have confirmed the marked increase in the incidence of opportunistic fungal infections, such as disseminated candidiasis and invasive aspergillosis. This increase is multifactorial in origin and reflects increased recognition as well as a growing population of patients at risk (ie, patients undergoing complex surgical procedures or intensive chemotherapy, as well as those

Table 1-1: Classification of Fungal Diseases Based on Location of Infection

- Systemic or deep mycoses—primarily involve internal organs and viscera
- Subcutaneous mycoses—infections of the subcutaneous tissue, fascia, or bone
- Cutaneous mycoses (dermatomycoses)—infections of the epidermis, hair, or nails

Table 1-2: Classification of Systemic Fungal Disorders in Humans

Group	Examples
The true molds–grow as molds in humans and in nature	*Aspergillus, Mucor* spp
The dimorphic fungi–grow as yeasts in humans and molds in nature	*Blastomyces dermatitidis* *Coccidioides immitis* *Histoplasma capsulatum* *Sporothrix schenckii*
The true yeasts–yeasts or yeast-like structures in humans and nature	*Cryptococcus neoformans* *Candida albicans*

with indwelling vascular devices). The rise in opportunistic fungal infections also reflects the improved survival of patients with underlying neoplasms, collagen vascular disease, and immunosuppression.

Traditionally, fungal infections are divided into three main groups: according to the site of infection (Table 1-1);

Table 1-3: Classification of Fungal Infections

Endemic (Sporadic) Mycoses

- Histoplasmosis–*Histoplasma capsulatum*
- Coccidioidomycosis–*Coccidioides immitis*
- Blastomycosis–*Blastomyces dermatitidis*
- Paracoccidioidomycosis–*Paracoccidioides brasiliensis*
- Sporotrichosis–*Sporothrix schenckii*

Opportunistic Mycoses

- Cryptococcosis
- Candidiasis
- Aspergillosis
- Zygomycosis
- Phaeohyphomycosis
- Hyalohyphomycosis

according to the type of fungus producing the infection, such as yeast, molds, or dimorphic fungi (Table 1-2); and according to whether fungal infections are endemic, such as histoplasmosis, or opportunistic, such as candidiasis (Table 1-3).

The purpose of this handbook is to provide a practical, authoritative reference that clinicians can use as a guide to diagnose and treat a wide variety of fungal infections.

Chapter **2**

Laboratory Diagnosis of Fungal Infections

The increase in the incidence of fungal infections has raised our awareness about the prevalence of mucosal and systemic fungal infections. It has also made us aware of the need to improve the diagnostic methods we use to identify a fungal infection.

These infections are associated with significant mortality and morbidity and are often not diagnosed, or are diagnosed late in the course of the disease, because current diagnostic techniques are less than ideal. Blood culture results are positive in only ~50% of cases of invasive candidiasis and in <5% of cases of invasive aspergillosis. Histopathologic diagnosis and cultures of samples obtained from protected anatomic sites are often not feasible in these critically ill populations; therefore, clinicians often face these diseases with little more than clinical and radiologic diagnostic clues. For these reasons, the development of new diagnostic methods have been a research priority in medical mycology.

Standard laboratory techniques to detect fungal elements in secretions and tissue include direct microscopic examination and several staining methods (Table 2-1).

The single best tool available for the diagnosis of fungal infections is the fungal culture (Table 2-2). Fungi can be cultured from the skin, mucosa, blood, tissues, and cerebrospinal fluid. In addition, serology may be useful for the

Table 2-1: Microscopic Examination for Fungi

Stained Smears of Exudates and Fluids

- Gram's stain
- Potassium hydroxide (KOH)
- Normal saline
- Giemsa stain
- Wright's stain

Wet Mounts—Unstained or With KOH

- Budding yeast cells—*Blastomyces dermatitidis* or *Candida* spp
- Budding cells with capsule—*Cryptococcus neoformans*
- Large cells with endospores—*Coccidioides immitis*
- Hyphae or broken fragments—*Aspergillus* spp, *Mucor* spp, *Rhizopus* spp

Special Stains of Tissues

- Hematoxylin-eosin (H&E)
  - Visualization of host tissue response
  - Hyaline or dematiaceous fungus?
- Gomori's methenamine silver (GMS)
  - One of the best screening stains, stains organisms black
- Periodic acid-Schiff (PAS)
  - Stains purulent exudates and organisms red
  - Best stain for internal structures
- PAS-Gridley
  - Stains background yellow, organisms red
- Mayer's mucicarmine stain
  - Stains capsule of *Cryptococcus* red
- Immunofluorescence (fluorescent antibody)

Table 2-2: Diagnosis of Systemic Fungal Disease

- Culture—best single tool
- Smear of body fluids and tissues—stained or unstained (wet prep)
- Skin test—coccidioidin (or spherulin) antigen is useful in some patients
- Histopathology and special stains of biopsy specimens
- Serology—only moderately helpful; especially the endemic fungi, cross-reactions, and false negatives

diagnosis of certain fungal diseases, including histoplasmosis and cryptococcosis. Although not readily available, polymerase chain reaction assays using broad-spectrum primers and nested primers appear to be able to identify fungal DNA despite negative cultures.

Among the new diagnostic techniques is the assay for the serum (1,3)-β-D-glucan (BG) derived from fungal cell walls. BG produced by fungi is detected by a glucan assay on the basis of its recognition by the innate immune system of horseshoe crabs, specifically *Tachypleus tridentatus* and *Limulus polyphemus*. Although this system is best known because of the activation of endotoxin from gram-negative bacteria by factor C zymogen, factor G zymogen is activated by BG, a substance that is present in many fungal cell walls. The *Limulus* amebocyte lysate (LAL) assay and the BG-specific variant Fungitell Assay (Associates of Cape Cod) are now approved for clinical use. This assay is manufactured by removing bacterial endotoxin-sensitive factor C from LAL, making this reagent specific for BG. This modified lysate is formulated with a synthetic chromogenic substrate and salts. The reagent is used in a quantitative assay that detects BG in the serum of patients with symptoms of invasive fungal infections. BG levels measured with a similar reagent prepared from *Tachypleus* have also proven to be highly sensitive and specific for BG in earlier clinical studies involving both candidiasis and human populations with a variety of fungal infections.

In a multicenter study published by Ostrosky-Zeichner, et al, the study group evaluated the assay as an aid to diagnosis of fungal infections. Subjects at four clinical sites in the United States were enrolled as either fungal infection-negative subjects (n = 170) or subjects with proven or probable IFI (n = 163). A central laboratory and four sites performed assays. A single sample was obtained per patient and was evaluated using an assay to detect serum BG derived from fungal cell walls (range 0 to >7,000 pg/mL).

At a cutoff of 60 pg/mL, the sensitivity and specificity of the assay were 69.9% and 87.1% respectively, with a positive predictive value (PPV) of 83.8% and a negative predictive value (NPV) of 75.1%. At a cutoff value of 80 pg/mL, the sensitivity and specificity were 64.4% and 92.4%, respectively, with a PPV of 89% and an NPV of 73%. Of the 107 patients with proven candidiasis, 81.3% had positive results at a cutoff value of 60 pg/mL, and 77.6% had positive results at a cutoff value of 80 pg/mL. Of the 10 patients with aspergillosis, 80% had positive results at cutoff values of 60 and 80 pg/mL. The three subjects diagnosed with *Fusarium* species had positive results at a cutoff value of 60 pg/mL. Patients infected with *Mucor* or *Rhizopus* species (both of which lack BG) had negative results at both cutoff values, and of the 12 patients with *Cryptococcus* infection, three had positive results at a cutoff value of 60 pg/mL, and two had positive results at a cutoff value of 80 pg/mL. Of the subjects with proven positive results who were receiving antifungal therapy (n = 118), 72.9% had results positive for BG at a cutoff value of 60 pg/mL, and 69.5% had results positive for BG at a cutoff value of 80 pg/mL.

Galactomannan is a cell wall polysaccharide that is released by *Aspergillus* species during growth. A commercially available sandwich ELISA (Platelia *Aspergillus*; BioRad) detects galactomannan by use of a monoclonal antibody which is used as both detector and captor. This antibody reacts with the (1,5)-β-linked galactofuranosyl residues that constitute the side chains of galactomannan. The test has been validated for serum specimens only and has a detection limit of ~1 ng/mL. Reported sensitivity and specificity range from 50% to 92.6% and from 94% to 99.6%, respectively, in patients with hematologic cancer. Reported positive and negative predictive values for patients with proven invasive aspergillosis range from 85% to 93% and 95% to 98.7%, respectively. False-positive results have been reported in adults and range from 5.7% to 14% when serum samples are used. Rates of false-positive results are higher among pediatric patients and neonates and may be as high as 83%. Reasons for false reactivity remain largely unknown, although recently, piperacillin/tazobactam (Zosyn®IV) was shown to cause cross-reactivity in adults, and cross-reacting epitopes from *Bifidobacterium* species were proposed as a cause in neonates.

Circulating galactomannan may be detected at a median of 5 to 8 days (range, 1 to 27 days) before clinical signs and symptoms of invasive aspergillosis become evident. Furthermore, the concentration of circulating galactomannan corresponds with the fungal tissue burden and may, therefore, be used to monitor the patient's response to antifungal treatment. Other methods to detect galactomannan include EIAs, RIAs, and latex agglutination tests. Only the latex agglutination test (Pastorex *Aspergillus*, BioRad) is commercially available and has a higher detection limit than the Platelia ELISA (15 ng/mL vs 1 ng/mL).

Because galactomannan is a water-soluble carbohydrate, it can also be detected in samples of other fluids, including urine and BAL. Although the Platelia ELISA is not validated for detection of galactomannan in these fluids, there is an increased tendency to use samples of these fluids, in addition to serum, for diagnosis of invasive aspergillosis.

The detection of galactomannan in specimens other than serum may provide additional evidence for invasive aspergillosis via a non-invasive method and may help to exclude false-positive or false-negative test results obtained using serum samples.

Invasive mycosis has become extremely common because of the increasing number of compromised hosts. Despite the availability of new and more potent antifungal agents, mortality rates remain high and have not decreased. The reason for this is because current diagnostic assays are not sensitive enough to detect early invasive fungal infections. For these reasons, the investigation and development of new diagnostic assays should be a priority.

Suggested Readings

Klont RR, Mennink-Kersten MA, Verweij PE: Utility of *Aspergillus* antigen detection in specimens other than serum specimens. *Clin Infect Dis* 2004;39:1467-1464.

Ostrosky-Zeichner L, Alexander BD, Kett DH, et al: Multicenter clinical evaluation of the (1,3) β-D-Glucan assay as an aid to diagnosis of fungal infections in humans. *Clin Infect Dis* 2005;41: 654-659.

Viscoli C, Machetti M, Cappellano P, et al: False-positive galactomannan Platelia *Aspergillus* test results for patients receiving piperacillin-tazobactam. *Clin Infect Dis* 2004;38:913-916.

Chapter 3

Amphotericin B

A lipophilic, polyene antifungal first isolated in 1955, amphotericin B has been available for clinical use since 1960 in a colloidal suspension, with deoxycholate as the solubilizing agent (Table 3-1).

Mechanism of action: Amphotericin B (Amphocin®, Fungizone®) exerts its antifungal effect by binding to ergosterol in the fungal cytoplasmic membrane, increasing permeability and causing leakage of intracellular components. Membrane channel activity is increased at lower doses, and pores are formed at higher concentrations.

Spectrum of activity: Amphotericin B exhibits broad-spectrum in vitro activity, including against most *Candida* species, except *C lusitaniae*. Occasionally, *C guilliermondii* and, rarely, *C parapsilosis* have been found to be resistant. It also has activity against *Histoplasma capsulatum*, *Coccidioides immitis*, *Blastomyces dermatitidis*, *Cryptococcus neoformans*, *Aspergillus fumigatus*, *Mucor* species, *Rhizopus* species, *Paracoccidioides brasiliensis*, *Sporothrix schenckii*, and *Rhodotorula* species.

Formulations: Amphotericin B is available in a powder for injection 50 mg; lozenges 10 mg; oral suspension 100 mg/mL; and a 3% cream, lotion, and ointment.

Dosages: The dosage is 0.7 to 1.5 mg/kg/d IV infused in 5% dextrose over 2 to 4 h; 10-mg lozenges; or 1 mL of a 100-mg/mL suspension PO q.i.d. Bladder irrigations in concentrations of 5 to 50 mg/mL of amphotericin B should be given for 3 days. The total dose of parenteral

Table 3-1: Classification of Antifungals

- **Polyenes**
  - Amphotericin B (Amphocin®, Fungizone®)
  - Amphotericin B lipid formulations (Abelcet®, AmBisome®, Amphotec®)
- **Flucytosine (Ancobon®)**
  - Adjunct to amphotericin B
- **Azoles**
  - Fluconazole (Diflucan®), itraconazole (Sporanox®)
  - Voriconazole (Vfend®), posaconazole (Noxafil®)
- **Echinocandins**
  - Caspofungin (Cancidas®), micafungin (Mycamine®), anidulafungin (Eraxis™)

amphotericin B must be adjusted based on the type of fungal infection being treated. Most patients receive a total dose of 0.5 to 1.5 g.

Pharmacokinetics: Amphotericin B is poorly absorbed; the metabolic pathways are unclear, but hepatic clearance is presumed, with 2% to 5% excreted unchanged in the urine. It is not removed by dialysis. Its initial serum half-life is 24 h, with a second-phase half-life of approximately 14 days.

Interactions: Concomitant administration of nephrotoxic antibiotics or nephrotoxic immunosuppressants, cyclosporine, or parenteral pentamidine (Nebupent®, Pentam®) may lead to an increased risk of nephrotoxicity. Amphotericin B may enhance the effects of neuromuscular blocking drugs and may increase the toxicity of digitalis glycosides.

Pregnancy: Amphotericin B is listed as a category B drug. Although usually safe, the drug's benefits should outweigh the risks.

Adverse events: Infusion-related toxicity occasionally occurs in the form of acute reactions 30 to 45 minutes after beginning infusion. Typically, chills, fever, and tachypnea may occur. Premedication with acetaminophen or the addition of hydrocortisone (25 to 50 mg) to the infusion solution may diminish reactions. Meperidine may be used to shorten rigors. Nephrotoxicity occurs in 30% to 40% of patients receiving parenteral amphotericin B. Patients should be monitored for changes in renal function (blood urea nitrogen, serum creatinine). Nephrotoxicity may be decreased by administering 0.5 to 1 L of 0.9% normal saline 1 to 2 h before each infusion. Electrolyte abnormalities include the depletion of potassium and magnesium, which occurs in almost 100% of patients.

Liver function test abnormalities include elevated transaminases (AST, ALT) in about 10% of patients. Thrombocytopenia and normocytic normochromic anemia are usually detected after 7 to 10 days of therapy. If therapy lasts more than 1 week, it is essential to monitor complete blood count with differential 3 times/week while the patient is on therapy.

Contraindications: Amphotericin B is contraindicated in patients with a hypersensitivity to the drug.

Indications: Amphotericin B is indicated for treatment of systemic fungal infections caused by susceptible organisms, fungal meningitis (cryptococcal meningitis, coccidioidal meningitis), cutaneous and mucocutaneous candidal infections, and candidal cystitis (IV or irrigation).

Suggested Readings

Barriere SL: Pharmacology and pharmacokinetics of traditional systemic antifungal agents. *Pharmacotherapy* 1990;10:134S-140S.

Chapman SW, Cleary JD, Rodgers PD: Amphotericin B. In: Dismukes WE, Pappas PG, Sobel JD, eds. *Clinical Mycology*, 1st ed. New York, NY, Oxford University Press, 2003, pp 33-48.

Gallis HA, Drew RH, Pickard WW: Amphotericin B: 30 years of clinical experience. *Rev Infect Dis* 1990;12:308-328.

Ghannoum MA, Rice LB: Antifungal agents: mode of action, mechanism of resistance, and correlation of these mechanisms with bacterial resistance. *Clin Microbiol Rev* 1999;12:501-517.

Rex JH, Stevens DA: Systemic antifungal agents. In: Mandell GL, Bennett JE, Dolin R, eds. *Principles and Practice of Infectious Diseases*, 6th ed. New York, NY, Churchill Livingstone, 2005 pp 502-513.

Chapter **4**

Lipid Formulations of Amphotericin B

Three amphotericin B lipid preparations (Amphotec®, Abelcet®, AmBisome®) have been approved by the US Food and Drug Administration (FDA). All appear to deliver higher concentrations of the drug with a theoretic increase in therapeutic potential and a decrease in nephrotoxicity. The three formulations include amphotericin B lipid complex (ABLC; Abelcet®); amphotericin B colloidal dispersion or amphotericin B cholesteryl sulfate complex

Table 4-1: Comparison of Amphotericin B Lipid Formulations in Relation to Amphotericin B Deoxycholate

Formulation	Nephrotoxicity	Infusion-related Adverse Events
Amphotericin B colloidal dispersion (Amphotec®)	↓	↔
Amphotericin B lipid complex (Abelcet®)	↓↓	↓
Liposomal amphotericin B (AmBisome®)	↓↓↓	↓↓

(ABCD; Amphotec®); and liposomal amphotericin B (L-AMB; AmBisome®). Although all are lipid preparations of amphotericin B, the different formulations are not interchangeable, and dosages may vary.

Formulations: ABCD comes in 50 mg/20 mL and 100 mg/50 mL vials; ABLC comes in 100 mg/20 mL vials; and L-AMB comes in 50 mg vials.

Dosages: ABCD, 3 to 6 mg/kg/d IV; ABLC, 3 to 5 mg/kg/d IV; L-AMB, 3 to 7 mg/kg/d IV.

Pharmacokinetics: ABCD distribution is multicompartmental; steady state increases with increasing dosage, possibly because of uptake from tissues. The serum half-life is 27 to 29 h. The drug is not removed by dialysis. ABLC is well distributed in the tissues, and the distribution volume increases with increasing doses. Although it is rapidly cleared from the bloodstream, it has a long terminal half-life of approximately 173 h because of the slow elimination from the tissues. Infusion of L-AMB results in a higher area under the curve (AUC) than is achieved with either conventional amphotericin B or the other lipid formula-

CNS Penetration	Electrolyte Disturbances	Cardiopulmonary Adverse Events
↔	↔	↑
↓	↓	↑
↓	↓↓	↑↑↑

Table 4-2: Characteristics of Lipid Preparations of Amphotericin B

Characteristics	ABLC
Formulation	Ribbons/sheets
Sterol	None
Lipid	DMPC, DMPG
Size (nm)	1,600 - 11,000
Half-life	173.4 h
FDA indications	Fungal infections refractory/intolerant to amphotericin B
Serum concentrations	
Peak (μg/mL)	1.7
Trough (μg/mL)	0.7
Area Under the Curve	17 μg/mL/h
Dosage	5 mg/kg/d

PC= phosphatidylcholine; DSPG= distearoyl phosphatidylglycerol; DMPC= dimyristoyl phosphatidylcholine; DMPG= dimyristoyl phosphatidyl glycerol

tions. It is distributed extensively into tissues, especially the reticuloendothelial organs. Its initial half-life is 7 h, and its terminal half-life is 100 to 150 h.

Interactions: Antineoplastic agents may enhance the potential of amphotericin B for renal toxicity, bronchospasm, and hypotension. Corticosteroids, digitalis, and thiazides may potentiate hypokalemia. The risk of renal toxicity is increased with cyclosporine and aminoglycosides.

Precautions: Lipid formulations of amphotericin B should not be given with leukocyte transfusions because

ABLC	**L-AMB**
Lipid Disk Cholesteryl sulfate None	Unilamellar vesicles Cholesteryl sulfate PC, DSPG
125	80 - 120
28.5 h	6.8 h
Aspergillosis refractory/intolerant to amphotericin B	Fungal infections refractory/ intolerant to amphotericin B Empirical therapy in febrile neutropenics Visceral leishmaniasis
3.1	83 50
43 μg/mL/h	555 μg/mL/h
3-6 mg/kg/d	3-5 mg/kg/d

ABLC=amphotericin B lipid complex

L-AMB=liposomal amphotericin B

of reported acute pulmonary reactions such as pulmonary infiltrates and hypoxia.

Pregnancy: This is a category B drug, usually safe, but benefits should outweigh risks.

Adverse events: The adverse side effects of lipid formulations of amphotericin B (Table 4-1) include nephrotoxicity, which, although considerably less than with desoxycholate (d)-amphotericin B, occurs in 15% to 25% of patients. Daily monitoring is required of blood urea nitrogen, serum creatinine, potassium, and magnesium levels. AmBisome® appears to have the best renal-sparing profile as well as an improved safety profile regarding infusion toxicity. Infusion-related toxicity includes fever, chills, rigors, nausea, vomiting, hypertension, tachycardia, and hypoxia. Elevated hepatic transaminases, alkaline phosphatases, and serum bilirubin may occur.

Indications: Lipid formulations of amphotericin B have FDA approval for treatment of adults and children with fungal infections. Abelcet® is indicated for the treatment of invasive fungal infections in patients who are refractory to or intolerant of conventional amphotericin B. AmBisome® is indicated for the treatment of cryptococcal meningitis in HIV infected patients; as empiric therapy for presumed fungal infections in febrile neutropenic patients; for the treatment of patients with aspergillosis, candidiasis, or cryptococcal infections refractory to conventional amphotericin B; or for patients in whom renal impairment or unacceptable toxicity precludes the use of conventional amphotericin B. AmBisome® is also approved for aspergillosis, candidiasis, and cryptococcosis and for empirical therapy of patients who are persistently febrile and neutropenic. These lipid formulations are indicated for any condition for which d-amphotericin B is indicated, particularly in patients who are at risk for nephrotoxicity.

Suggested Readings

Chapman SW, Cleary JD, Rodgers PD: Amphotericin B. In: Dismukes WE, Pappas PG, Sobel JD, eds. *Clinical Mycology*, 1st ed. New York, NY, Oxford University Press, 2003, pp 33-48.

Rex JH, Stevens DA: Systemic antifungal agents. In: Mandell GL, Bennett JE, Dolin R, eds. *Principles and Practice of Infectious Diseases*, 6th ed. New York, NY, Churchill Livingstone, 2005 pp 502-513.

Wong-Beringer A, Jacobs RA, Guglielmo BJ: Lipid formulations of amphotericin B: clinical efficacy and toxicities. *Clin Infect Dis* 1998;27:603-618.

Chapter 5

Nystatin

Nystatin (Mycostatin®) is a polyene antifungal obtained from *Streptomyces noursei*.

Mechanism of action: Nystatin exerts its antifungal effect by binding to ergosterol in the fungal cytoplasmic membrane, increasing permeability and causing leakage of intracellular components. Membrane channel activity is increased at lower doses, and pores are formed at higher concentrations.

Spectrum of activity: Nystatin exhibits broad-spectrum in vitro activity, including against most *Candida* species, *Histoplasma capsulatum*, *Coccidioides immitis*, *Blastomyces dermatitidis*, *Cryptococcus neoformans*, *Aspergillus fumigatus*, *Mucor* species, *Rhizopus* species, *Paracoccidioides brasiliensis*, *Sporothrix schenckii*, and *Rhodotorula* species.

Formulations: Nystatin comes in tablets 500,000 U; suspension 100,000 U/mL; powder for suspension 50 million U, 150 million U, and 500 million U; vaginal suppositories 100,000 U; cream, ointment, and powder 100,000 U/g; and lozenges 200,000 U.

Dosages: Vaginal candidiasis, 100,000 U vaginal tab, dissolve 1 tab qhs for 14 days. Oropharyngeal candidiasis, 400,000 to 600,000 U of oral suspension q.i.d. swish and swallow for 7 to 14 days; 200,000 U lozenges, dissolve 1 to 2 pastilles 4 to 5 times daily for 7 to 14 days.

Pharmacokinetics: Nystatin is not absorbed from any surface, so there is no detectable amount in the body. No interactions have been reported.

Pregnancy: Nystatin is a category B drug, safe in pregnancy.

Adverse events: Gastrointestinal effects include nausea, vomiting, and diarrhea.

Precautions: Nystatin should not be used to treat systemic mycoses, and it is ineffective in systemic fungal infections.

Indications: Nystatin is indicated for oropharyngeal candidiasis, for cutaneous or mucocutaneous candidal infections, and for selected patients with vaginitis caused by non-*albicans Candida* species.

Suggested Reading

Chapman SW, Cleary JD, Rodgers PD: Amphotericin B. In: Dismukes WE, Pappas PG, Sobel JD, eds. *Clinical Mycology*, 1st ed. New York, NY, Oxford University Press, 2003, pp 33-48.

Rex JH, Stevens DA: Systemic antifungal agents. In: Mandell GL, Bennett JE, Dolin R, eds. *Principles and Practice of Infectious Diseases*, 6th ed. New York, NY, Churchill Livingstone, 2005 pp 502-513.

Chapter 6

Flucytosine

Flucytosine (5-FC, Ancobon®) is a water-soluble, fluorinated pyrimidine analog.

Mechanism of action: Flucytosine is converted to fluorouracil after penetrating fungal cells. It inhibits RNA and protein synthesis. It is generally used in combination with amphotericin B and rarely used as a single agent because of the ability of organisms to quickly develop resistance in vivo.

Spectrum of activity: Flucytosine exhibits in vitro activity against most strains of *Candida* and *Cryptococcus*.

Formulations: Flucytosine is available in 250-mg and 500-mg capsules.

Dosage: 100 to 150 mg/kg/d divided q 6 h orally.

Pharmacokinetics: The bioavailability of flucytosine is 75% to 90%. It has a wide distribution in many tissues throughout the body. Cerebrospinal fluid levels vary from 60% to 100% of serum levels. Only small amounts are metabolized in the body, while 75% to 90% of the drug is excreted unchanged in the urine. The serum half-life is approximately 2 to 6 h with normal renal function.

Interactions: There is possible enhanced toxicity with the coadministration of amphotericin B because of decreased renal function associated with amphotericin B use.

Pregnancy: Flucytosine is a category C drug; its safety for use during pregnancy has not been established.

Adverse events: The overall toxicity of flucytosine is approximately 30%. Dosage adjustment is required to produce a plasma concentration of 25 to 50 μg/mL. The adverse event of greatest concern is myelosuppression (22%), especially neutropenia, which is associated with blood concentrations of >125 μg/mL. Dosage needs to be adjusted in renal impairment. Allopurinol can minimize the myelosuppressive effect. Other adverse events include renal insufficiency, diarrhea, nausea, vomiting, and elevated AST and ALT. Patchy hepatic necrosis has been reported rarely.

Precautions: Monitor complete blood count with differential, renal function, and hepatic function 3 times/week. Use cautiously in patients with underlying renal insufficiency, hepatic failure, or bone marrow suppression.

Indications: Flucytosine is indicated in severe fungal infections caused by susceptible strains of *Candida* and *Cryptococcus* and in chromoblastomycosis, but it is rarely used as monotherapy. It is generally used in combination with amphotericin B because of limited data demonstrating synergistic activity and because of the rapid development of resistance when it is used alone. Most common indications include cryptococcal meningitis and *Candida* endocarditis and meningitis. Also, high urine concentrations make flucytosine useful in treating symptomatic candiduria, especially in the presence of *C glabrata*.

Suggested Readings

Barriere SL: Pharmacology and pharmacokinetics of traditional systemic antifungal agents. *Pharmacotherapy* 1990;10:134S-140S.

Ghannoum MA, Rice LB: Antifungal agents: mode of action, mechanism of resistance, and correlation of these mechanisms with bacterial resistance. *Clin Microbiol Rev* 1999;12:501-517.

Larsen RA: Flucytosine. In: Dismukes WE, Pappas PG, Sobel JD, eds. *Clinical Mycology*. 1st ed. New York, NY, Oxford University Press, 2003, pp 59-63.

Rex JH, Stevens DA: Systemic antifungal agents. In: Mandell GL, Bennett JE, Dolin R, eds. *Principles and Practice of Infectious Diseases*, 6th ed. New York, NY, Churchill Livingstone, 2005, pp 502-513.

Chapter 7

Azoles

The azoles are synthetic antifungal compounds that fall into two groups, imidazoles and triazoles. Triazoles have three atoms of nitrogen in the azole ring, while imidazoles have only two atoms of nitrogen in the azole ring. Imidazole agents include miconazole, ketoconazole, butoconazole, tioconazole, econazole, terconazole, and clotrimazole. Triazole agents include fluconazole, itraconazole, voriconazole, and posaconazole (Table 7-1).

Topical agents may be used to manage local forms of candidiasis such as cutaneous candidiasis, oropharyngeal candidiasis, esophageal candidiasis, and vulvovaginal candidiasis. These preparations are available as creams for topical use, as troches for oropharyngeal candidiasis, and as vaginal suppositories or tablets for vaginitis. Agents used to treat systemic fungal infections are available in various oral and injectable forms, described below.

The primary mechanism of action of the azoles is inhibition of cytochrome P-450-dependent lanosterol 14-α-demethylase, an enzyme required for the synthesis of ergosterol, the main component of fungal cell membranes. This results in the accumulation of methylated sterols, depletion of ergosterol, and inhibition of cell growth.

Ketoconazole

Ketoconazole (Nizoral®) is an orally active imidazole that was approved in 1981. For many years, ketoconazole was the only available oral antifungal agent for the treatment of serious fungal infections.

Table 7-1: Azole Antifungals

Systemic Azoles

- Ketoconazole (Nizoral®)
- Fluconazole (Diflucan®)
- Itraconazole (Sporanox®)
- Voriconazole (Vfend®)
- Posaconazole (Noxafil®)

Topical Azoles

- Miconazole (Monistat®)
- Clotrimazole (Lotrimin®, Mycelex®)
- Butoconazole (Femstat 3®, Gynazole-1®)
- Tioconazole (Vagistat-1®)
- Terconazole (Terazol® 3, Terazol® 7)
- Econazole (Spectazole®)
- Sulconazole (Exelderm®)
- Oxiconazole (Oxistat®)

Spectrum of activity: Ketoconazole is active in vitro against *Cryptococcus neoformans*, most *Candida* species, *Coccidioides immitis*, *Histoplasma capsulatum*, *Blastomyces dermatitidis*, *Sporothrix schenckii*, *Paracoccidioides brasiliensis*, and a variety of dermatophytes.

Formulations: Ketoconazole is available in 200-mg tablets and 2% cream and shampoo.

Dosage: For severe fungal infections, the dosage is 200 mg/d, which may be increased to 400 mg/d if no response. The topical preparation is applied to the affected area twice daily for 2 to 6 weeks. The shampoo is applied twice weekly for 4 weeks.

Pediatric dosage: For children 2 years of age and older, the dosage is 3.3 to 6.6 mg/kg/d.

Pharmacokinetics: Ketoconazole is converted to the hydrochloride salt before absorption. Absorption may be erratic and is decreased by increases in gastric pH. The bioavailability of ketoconazole appears to be about 75%. Once absorbed, the drug is metabolized by the liver and is excreted as inactive metabolites in the bile and feces.

Interactions: Ketoconazole absorption is decreased by drugs that elevate gastric pH, such as antacids and histamine H_2-receptor blockers. Ketoconazole may increase serum levels of warfarin, cyclosporine, phenytoin, and sulfonylureas. Rifampin (Rifadin®, Rifadin®IV)and phenytoin may decrease levels of ketoconazole. Concomitant alcohol use may cause a disulfiram-like reaction.

Adverse events: The common side effects of ketoconazole are nausea, vomiting, and anorexia, which are dose limiting. But the most serious side effect of ketoconazole is hepatotoxicity, at a rate of about 1 in 10,000 cases. Hepatotoxicity is the single complication that reduces the widespread use of ketoconazole. In addition, ketoconazole also blocks adrenal steroid synthesis and has antiandrogenic properties that produce impotence, decreased libido, and gynecomastia in men and menstrual irregularities and alopecia in women.

Contraindications: Ketoconazole should not be used with cisapride or with astemizole because of potential cardiovascular toxicity, and it should not be used with alcohol because of a disulfiram-like reaction. It should be used cautiously in patients with hepatic disease.

Pregnancy: Ketoconazole is a category C agent; its safety for use in pregnancy has not been established.

Indications: For many years, ketoconazole was the drug of choice for a variety of fungal infections, including histoplasmosis; blastomycosis; coccidioidomycosis; paracoccidioidomycosis; chronic mucocutaneous candidiasis; oropharyngeal, esophageal, and vaginal candidiasis; tinea; and seborrheic dermatitis. Because of the recent discovery and production of safer triazoles (fluconazole and itraconazole), which have fewer adverse events and improved efficacy, ketoconazole is no longer the drug of choice for most of these infections.

Fluconazole

Fluconazole (Diflucan®) is a water-soluble, broad-spectrum triazole that was approved in 1990. Fluconazole has substantially less effect on human sterol metabolism than the older azoles and so has fewer adverse events than those azoles.

Spectrum of activity: Fluconazole is active in vitro against *C neoformans*, *Candida* species (except *Candida krusei*), *C immitis*, *H capsulatum*, *B dermatitidis*, and a variety of dermatophytes (Table 7-2).

Formulations: Fluconazole is available in 50-mg, 100-mg, 150-mg, and 200-mg tablets; in 10 mg/mL and 40 mg/mL suspensions; and in a 200 mg/100 mL or 400 mg/200 mL injection.

Dosage: For oropharyngeal and esophageal candidiasis, the recommended dose of fluconazole is 200 mg on day 1, followed by 100 mg/d for at least 2 weeks after resolution of symptoms. For vaginal candidiasis, 150 mg oral single dose; for systemic candidiasis or candidemia, 800 mg on day 1 as the loading dose, followed by 400 mg/d IV or PO to be continued for at least 2 weeks after blood cultures have cleared or symptoms have resolved. If blood culture is positive for *Candida* (*Torulopsis*) *glabrata*, the fluconazole daily dose should be increased to 800 mg/d. For acute cryptococcal meningitis (mild to moderate), the dose should be 800 mg on day 1, followed by 400 mg/d for at least 10 to 12 weeks after cerebrospinal fluid (CSF) cultures become negative. For suppressive therapy of cryptococcal disease after initial acute treatment in HIV-positive patients, fluconazole 200 mg/d is recommended for life. For candiduria, fluconazole 200 mg/d is recommended for at least 2 weeks; for prophylaxis in patients undergoing bone marrow transplant, 400 mg/d starting several days before neutropenia and at least 1 week after absolute neutrophil count rises above 1,000 cells/mm^3.

Pediatric dosage: For children older than 4 weeks, 3 mg/kg/d for superficial infections and 6 to 12 mg/kg/d for systemic infections. For infants younger than 2 weeks, doses should be administered q 72 h.

Pharmacokinetics: After oral administration, absorption of fluconazole is rapid and complete, with bioavailability >90%. The drug is well distributed throughout the body and is partially metabolized in the liver. Excretion is primarily via the kidneys, where more than 80% is excreted unchanged in the urine. Excretion rate depends on renal function (Table 7-3).

Interactions: Fluconazole levels may increase with hydrochlorothiazide but may decrease (30%) with the coadministration of rifampin. The coadministration of fluconazole may increase concentrations of phenytoin, theophylline, tolbutamide, glyburide, glipizide, cyclosporine, terfenadine, astemizole, cisapride, and tacrolimus (Prograf®, Protopic®); effects of anticoagulants may increase with fluconazole coadministration.

Adverse events: Nausea, vomiting, diarrhea, and allergic reactions are the most common adverse effects. Clinicians should monitor patients closely for the development of rashes (10%) and discontinue fluconazole if lesions progress or if there are elevated transaminases (10%). Clinical hepatitis with cholestasis and fulminant hepatic failure (including death) has occurred rarely. Fluconazole is not recommended during breast-feeding.

Precautions: Dosage adjustment for renal insufficiency is recommended. If the creatinine clearance is between 25 and 49 mL/min, the dose should be decreased by 50%; if it is <25 mL/min, the dose should be decreased by 75%.

Table 7-2: Azole Antifungal Spectrum of Activity

Organism	Fluconazole
Yeast	
C albicans	++
Flu/Itra resistant	–
C glabrata	–/+
C krusei	–
C tropicalis	+
C parapsilosis	++
C lusitaniae	++
Cryptococcus neoformans	++
Trichosporon ashaii	+/++
Dimorphic fungi	
Blastomyces dermatitidis	+
Histoplasma capsulatum	+
Coccidioides immitis	+
Sporothrix schenckii	+
Paracoccidioides brasiliensis	+

\+ Moderate activity in vitro and/or in animals models

++ Excellent activity in vitro and/or in animal model

In patients on hemodialysis, the usual daily dose should be given after each dialysis session.

Pregnancy: Fluconazole is a category C agent; its safety for use during pregnancy has not been established.

Itraconazole	Voriconazole	Posaconazole
++	++	++
–/+	+	+
–/+	+	+
–/+	++	+
++	++	++
++	++	++
++	++	++
+/++	++	++
++	++	++
++	+/++	++
++	++	++
+	+	+
++	+	++
++	NA	++

– No clinically useful activity

NA, not available

(continued on next page)

Indications: Fluconazole is indicated for oropharyngeal, esophageal, and vaginal candidiasis; candidemia and invasive candidiasis; candiduria; fungal prophylaxis in bone marrow transplant patients; acute therapy for mild to

Table 7-2: Azole Antifungal Spectrum of Activity *(continued)*

Organism	Fluconazole
Molds	
Aspergillus fumigatus	–
Aspergillus flavus	–
Aspergillus terreus	–
Fusarium solani	–
Rhizopus sp	–
Mucor sp	–
Scedosporium apiospermum	+
Scedosporium prolificans	–
Dematiaceous fungi	–

+ Moderate activity in vitro and/or in animals models

++ Excellent activity in vitro and/or in animal model

moderate cryptococcal meningitis; and suppressive therapy of cryptococcal meningitis in patients with AIDS.

Itraconazole

Itraconazole (Sporanox®) is a synthetic, lipophilic triazole that has less effect on human sterol metabolism and does not decrease cortisol or testosterone levels as ketoconazole does. It has fewer adverse effects than the older systemic imidazoles.

Spectrum of activity: Itraconazole in vitro exhibits activity against a broad spectrum of fungi, including *C albicans* and many non-*albicans Candida* species,

Itraconazole	Voriconazole	Posaconazole
+	++	++
++	++	++
++	+	++
–	–/+	–/+
–/+	–	+
–/+	–	–
+	+/++	+/++
–	–/+	–
+/++	+/++	+/++

– No clinically useful activity

NA, not available

C neoformans, *C immitis*, *H capsulatum*, *P brasiliensis*, *B dermatitidis*, *S schenckii*, *Aspergillus* species, and a variety of dermatophytes.

Formulations: Itraconazole is supplied as 100-mg capsules, a 10 mg/mL oral solution, and a 10 mg/mL injection. The oral solution and injection contain itraconazole solubilized by hydroxypropyl-β-cyclodextrin as a molecular inclusion complex.

Dosage: For cutaneous candidiasis and onychomycosis, the dosage should be 200 mg b.i.d. for 7 days/month for 3 to 6 months; for oropharyngeal and esophageal candidiasis, 200 mg/d IV/PO for 7 to 14 days after resolution of symp-

Table 7-3: Pharmacokinetics of Azole Antifungals

Parameter	Fluconazole
Bioavailability (%)	>90
Fasting	
Effect of food on bioavailability	No effect
Time to peak concentration (hours)	1-2
Peak concentration (μg/mL)	
at steady state:	3.86-4/07
IV (dosage)	100 mg daily
Oral (dosage)	4.1-8.1 (400 g x 1)
Tissue penetration (% simultaneous serum)	
CSF	50-94
Lung	100
Protein binding (%)	11-12
Elimination half-life (hours)	22-31
% Unchanged drug in urine	80

CSF = cerebrospinal fluid; NA = Data not available.
*Absolute oral bioavailability is not known because of the absence of parenteral dosage form. Value represents bioavailability relative to oral solution.

**Oral bioavailability depends on dosage form. Higher values represent data from commercially available oral solution when given to healthy volunteers.

***Human data not available. Values represent data from animal studies.

Itraconazole	Voriconazole	Posaconazole
55-> 90**	≥90	8-47***
See text	Decreased	Increased
4-5	1-3	3
2.9 [1.9]† (22 mg b.i.d. x 2, then 200 mg daily x 5)	3.00 (3 mg/kg/b.i.d.)	NA
2.0-2.3 [2.1-2.6] (200 mg b.i.d.)	1.9 (200 mg b.i.d.)	1.1 (200 mg b.i.d.)
< 1	42-67	NA
100	NA	NA
99.8 [99.5]†	58	NA
38-64†† [27-57]†	6†	24
< 1	< 5	Minimal

†Values in brackets are parameters for hydroxyitraconazole.
††Dose-dependent elimination has been reported. Values may be higher or lower depending on dosage.

toms; for blastomycosis, histoplasmosis, and aspergillosis, 100 to 200 mg PO twice daily. For severe, life-threatening infections, the loading dose is 200 mg t.i.d. for the first 3 days, followed by 200 mg b.i.d.

Pediatric dosage: For cutaneous candidiasis in pediatric patients, the dosage should be 3 to 5 mg/kg/d for 30 days.

Pharmacokinetics: Oral bioavailability of itraconazole capsules is maximized when they are taken with food and gastric pH is acidic; bioavailability is approximately 55%. The bioavailability of the oral solution is 55%, which is increased by the fasting state to almost 100%. Itraconazole is extensively distributed into tissues, especially the lungs, brain, kidneys, liver, spleen, bone, and muscle, where the drug concentrations are two to three times higher than the corresponding plasma concentration. Itraconazole is metabolized by the liver into many metabolites, including hydroxyitraconazole, the major metabolite that possesses in vitro activity similar to the parent compound. Renal excretion of parent drug is <1%; about 40% of the dose is excreted as inactive metabolites in urine.

Interactions: Antacids may reduce absorption of itraconazole. Edema may occur with coadministration of calcium channel blockers (eg, amlodipine [Norvasc®], nifedipine [Adalat® CC]). Itraconazole may decrease the elimination of drugs metabolized by CYP3A4, while inducers of 3A4 may decrease plasma concentrations of itraconazole, and inhibitors may increase levels of itraconazole (Table 7-4). Rhabdomyolysis has been reported with the coadministration of HMG CoA-reductase inhibitors (lovastatin [Mevacor®] or simvastatin [Zocor®]). Serious cardiovascular events—including QT prolongation, torsades de pointes, ventricular tachycardia, and sudden cardiac death—have occurred when itraconazole was given with cisapride, pimozide (Orap®), or quinidine.

Adverse events: Nausea, vomiting, diarrhea, and abdominal discomfort are common side effects. High doses may produce hypertension, hypokalemia, or edema.

Table 7-4: Itraconazole Drug Interactions

Drug Plasma Concentrations Increased by Itraconazole

- Digoxin
- Quinidine
- Carbamazepine
- Rifabutin
- Pimozide
- Long-acting barbiturates
- Cisapride
- Cyclosporine
- Tacrolimus
- Sirolimus

Drugs that Decrease Plasma Concentrations of Itraconazole

- Carbamazepine
- Phenytoin
- Rifampin

Precautions: Itraconazole should be used cautiously in patients with hepatic insufficiency. Liver function tests in patients with preexisting hepatic dysfunction should be monitored. Itraconazole should not be given to patients with creatinine clearance of <30 mL/min.

Contraindications: Itraconazole should not be used concomitantly with quinidine, dofetilide, pimozide, cisapride, or HMG CoA-reductase inhibitors.

Pregnancy: Itraconazole is a category C agent; its safety for use during pregnancy has not been established.

Indications: Itraconazole is indicated for cutaneous, oral, esophageal, and vaginal candidiasis; histoplasmosis, blastomycosis, sporotrichosis, and coccidioidomycosis; dermatophyte infections; and onychomycosis. It is also indicated for aspergillosis in patients who are intolerant of, or refractory to, amphotericin B therapy, as well as consolidation therapy in such patients following a course of amphotericin

B. Itraconazole is indicated as empirical therapy of febrile neutropenic patients with suspected fungal infections and as primary prophylaxis in neutropenic patients.

Voriconazole

Voriconazole (Vfend®), a new lipophilic triazole, was approved by the US Food and Drug Administration in 2002.

Spectrum of activity: Voriconazole exhibits in vitro activity against a broad range of fungi, including *C albicans*, non-*albicans Candida* species, *Aspergillus* species, *Fusarium* species, *Scedosporium apiospermum*, *Trichosporon* species, *Penicillium* species, *C neoformans*, *H capsulatum*, *B dermatitidis*, *C immitis*, *Paracoccidioides* species, and a variety of dermatophytes.

Formulations: Voriconazole is available in 50-mg and 200-mg tablets and a 200-mg vial for injection with 3.2 g sulfobutyl ether β-cyclodextrin (SBECD), and voriconazole oral suspension.

Dosage: A loading dose of 6 mg/kg q 12 h IV should be given for one day, followed by 4 mg/kg q 12 h IV. Orally, 400 mg PO q 12 h should be given for two doses, followed by 200 mg q 12 h.

Pharmacokinetics: The oral bioavailability of voriconazole is about 96% in the fasting state, with nonlinear kinetics from first-pass metabolism. The drug undergoes extensive hepatic metabolism by three cytochrome P-450 enzymes, CYP2C19, 2C9, and 3A4. Voriconazole is metabolized primarily via the liver and eliminated through the kidney, where <2% of the drug is excreted unchanged in the urine.

Interactions: Voriconazole may decrease the elimination of drugs metabolized by CYP3A4, while 3A4 inducers may decrease plasma concentrations of voriconazole and inhibitors of 3A4 may increase levels of voriconazole (Table 7-5). Hypoglycemia may occur with sulfonylureas. Voriconazole increases exposure to warfarin, sirolimus

Table 7-5: Voriconazole Drug Interactions

- Rifampin*, barbiturates† (long-acting), carbamazepine† (decreased voriconazole exposure)
- Sirolimus*, astemizole†, cisapride†, pimozide†, quinidine†, ergot alkaloids†
(voriconazole increases exposure to these medications)

* Interaction with these agents has been clinically studied.

† Interaction with these agents has not been studied but is suggested by their pharmacokinetics.

(Rapamune®), tacrolimus, astemizole, terfenadine, cisapride, pimozide, quinidine, ergot alkaloids, cyclosporine, digoxin, midazolam or triazolam (Halcion®), and phenytoin plasma concentrations. Coadministration with cisapride may cause cardiac rhythm abnormalities and death. Conversely, carbamazepine (Carbatrol®, Tegretol®, Tegretol®-XR), barbiturates, phenytoin, rifampin, and rifabutin (Mycobutin®) reduce voriconazole levels.

Precautions: Accumulation of the intravenous vehicle occurs in patients with moderate to severe renal dysfunction (creatinine clearance <50 mL/min). Oral voriconazole should be administered to these patients, unless an assessment of the benefits and risks to the patient justifies the use of intravenous voriconazole.

Contraindications: Voriconazole is contraindicated with rifampin, barbiturates (long-acting), sirolimus, terfenadine, astemizole, ergot alkaloids, carbamazepine, quinidine, pimozide, and cisapride.

Adverse events: In clinical trials, skin rashes related to voriconazole therapy were observed in 6% of patients. Elevations in AST, ALT, total bilirubin, and alkaline phosphatase have occurred in 4% to 20% of patients.

Transient visual disturbances occurred in about 24% of patients (363/1,493) enrolled in clinical trials and have been described as alterations in color or light, decreased vision, enhanced perception of light, blurred vision, and photophobia. Generally, these visual effects tend to occur with the first few doses of voriconazole; the onset is usually 30 to 60 minutes after the dose, and they last for 30 to 60 minutes. The cause of these visual abnormalities may be receptor de-excitation blockage in the retina by voriconazole. However, no residual sequelae have been described, and few patients (0.5%) have discontinued therapy because of these visual abnormalities.

Pregnancy: Voriconazole is a category D agent.

Indications: Voriconazole is approved as primary therapy for invasive aspergillosis, for disseminated fusariosis, and for infections due to *S apiospermum* (*Pseudallescheria boydii*), candidemia and disseminated candidiasis in non-neutropenic patients, and esophageal candidiasis. In addition, clinical trials have demonstrated voriconazole's ability to decrease the frequency of breakthrough fungal infections in febrile neutropenic patients.

Posaconazole

Posaconazole (Noxafil®) is a novel, synthetic, lipophilic triazole antifungal agent structurally similar to itraconazole. In addition, SCH-59884, a water-soluble prodrug of posaconazole, is being evaluated for intravenous use.

Spectrum of activity: Posaconazole in vitro exhibits activity against a broad range of fungi, including *C albicans*, non-*albicans Candida* species, *Aspergillus* species, *Fusarium* species, *S apiospermum*, *Trichosporon* species, *Penicillium* species, *C neoformans*, *H capsulatum*, *B dermatitidis*, *C immitis*, *P brasiliensis*, *Rhizopus* species, *Mucor* species, *Trypansoma cruzi*, and a variety of dermatophytes. It was shown to be efficacious in animal models of candidiasis, aspergillosis, blastomycosis, cryptococcosis, histoplasmosis, coccidioidomycosis, and *T cruzi* infection.

In preclinical, in vitro, and in vivo animal models, posaconazole displayed activity against a wide spectrum of fungi, including aspergillosis, fusarium, and zygomycetes.

Formulations: Posaconazole is available as an oral suspension containing 40 mg/mL.

Dosage: The dose depends on the indication. When used as prophylaxis for invasive fungal infections, the dose is 200 mg (5 mL) t.i.d.; for oropharyngeal candidiasis, the recommended dose is 100 mg (2.5 mL) b.i.d on day one, followed by 100 mg (2.5 mL) daily for 14 days; when used for refractory oropharyngeal candidiasis, the dose is 400 mg (10 mL) b.i.d.

Pharmacokinetics: The oral bioavailability of posaconazole is increased when taken with a high-fat meal (~50 g of fat) relative to when the drug is taken in a fasted state. The drug is primarily metabolized via UDP glucuronidation and is a substrate for P-glycoprotein efflux. It does not have any major circulating metabolites. Posaconazole has a half-life of 35 hours and is eliminated primarily in the feces. Renal clearance is minimal, with less than 15% of the dose excreted in the urine.

Interactions: Posaconazole is an inhibitor of CTP3A4. Coadministration of posaconazole with rifabutin, phenytoin, cimetidine, and efavirenz decreases the plasma concentration of posaconazole. The coadministration of posaconazole with sirolimus, cyclosporine, tacrolimus, midazolam, ritonavir, and atazanavir increases their serum concentrations.

Precautions: Posaconazole should be administered cautiously in patients with proarrhythmic conditions.

Contraindications: Posaconazole is contraindicated with sirolimus, with drugs that are known to prolong the QTc interval, and with drugs that are metabolized through CYP3A4.

Adverse events: In clinical trials, the most common side effects include abdominal pain, diarrhea, nausea, vomiting, rash, and liver enzyme abnormalities.

Pregnancy: Posaconazole is a category C.

Indications: Indicated for oropharyngeal candidiasis, oropharyngeal candidiasis refractory to itraconazole and/or fluconazole, and as prophylaxis of invasive fungal infections.

Miconazole

Miconazole (Monistat 3®, Monistat 7®, Monistat-Derm®, Micatin®, Femizol-M®) was the first available systemic imidazole antifungal agent. It was approved in 1978.

Spectrum of activity: Miconazole has in vitro activity against a broad range of fungi, including *C albicans*, non-*albicans Candida* species, *Aspergillus* species, *S apiospermum*, *Trichosporon* species, *C neoformans*, *H capsulatum*, *C immitis*, *P brasiliensis*, *S schenckii*, *Microsporum canis*, and *Curvularia* species.

Formulations: Miconazole is available by prescription as a 2% vaginal cream, a 2% topical cream, and a 200-mg vaginal suppository; it is available over the counter as a 2% powder, a 2% spray, and a 100-mg vaginal suppository. Because miconazole is poorly soluble, the IV form is administered in a lipid vehicle, which appears to be responsible for most adverse effects.

Dosage: For vaginal candidiasis: insert one 200-mg suppository intravaginally qhs for 3 days or one 100-mg vaginal suppository qhs for 7 days, or insert one applicator of vaginal cream qhs for 7 days. For topical use: apply to affected area b.i.d. for 2 to 4 weeks. If the cream is used, apply sparingly to avoid maceration effects. The parenteral dosage is 600 mg (over 30 to 60 min) t.i.d.

Pharmacokinetics: A small amount of miconazole is absorbed systemically via topical applications. Miconazole is metabolized in the liver to inactive compounds; most is excreted in feces (50%), while 10% to 22% is excreted in urine.

Interactions: No interactions have been reported with topical miconazole. Drug-drug interactions have not been well studied with the parenteral preparations; however, because of miconazole's structure and its interaction with the cytochrome P-450 system, clinicians must assume it has interactions similar to those of the other imidazoles, such as ketoconazole.

Precautions: Use only externally, avoid contact with eyes. Use cautiously in patients with hepatic insufficiency.

Adverse events: Topical preparation: occasional sensitivity or chemical irritation may occur. Parenteral preparation: a high frequency of side effects has been attributed to the lipid vehicle, including phlebitis, pruritus, nausea, vomiting, fever, chills, and anemia. Rapid infusion of the drug has led to cardiorespiratory arrest and anaphylactic reaction from massive histamine release.

Pregnancy: Miconazole is a category C agent; its safety for use during pregnancy has not been established.

Indications: The topical preparation of miconazole is indicated for cutaneous and mucosal fungal infections, including candidiasis and pityriasis versicolor. Because of its high incidence of toxicity and the availability of newer antifungals, parenteral miconazole is no longer needed.

Clotrimazole

Clotrimazole (FemCare®, Gyne-Lotrimin®, Lotrimin®, Lotrimin AF®, Mycelex®, Femizole-7®, Mycelex-G®, Mycelex-7®) is a synthetic, broad-spectrum topical imidazole.

Spectrum of activity: Clotrimazole has in vitro activity against a broad range of fungi, including *C albicans*, non-*albicans Candida* species, and several dermatophytes.

Formulations: Clotrimazole is available by prescription in the form of 100-mg, 200-mg, and 500-mg vaginal tablets; 1% topical cream, lotion, and solution; and 10-mg oral lozenges (troches). It is available without a prescription in the form of 100-mg vaginal tablets; 1% vaginal cream; and a combination pack of 500-mg vaginal tablets/1% topical cream.

Dosage: For oropharyngeal candidiasis: 10-mg troche dissolved in the mouth 5 times/day for 7 days. For cutaneous candidiasis: apply 1% cream, lotion, or solution b.i.d./t.i.d. for 1 to 8 weeks. For vaginal candidiasis: 100-mg vaginal tablets qd for 7 days or 1 applicator intravaginally of 1%, 2%, or 10% cream qhs for 7 to 14 days.

Pharmacokinetics: A small amount of clotrimazole is absorbed systemically via topical applications.

Interactions: None reported.

Adverse events: Clotrimazole occasionally produces nausea, vomiting, an unpleasant taste (lozenges), and vaginal burning and itching.

Precautions: None.

Pregnancy: Clotrimazole is a category B agent; it is usually safe, but the benefits must outweigh the risks.

Indications: Clotrimazole is indicated for cutaneous, oropharyngeal, and vaginal candidiasis; tinea pedis, tinea cruris, and tinea corporis; and pityriasis versicolor.

Butoconazole Nitrate

Butoconazole (Femstat 3®, Gynazole-1®) is a synthetic, broad-spectrum imidazole that comes in a topical preparation.

Spectrum of activity: Butoconazole has in vitro activity against a broad range of fungi, including *C albicans*, non-*albicans Candida* species, and several dermatophytes.

Formulations: Butoconazole is available over the counter as a 2% vaginal cream.

Dosage: For vaginal candidiasis: insert one applicator (5 g) intravaginally qhs for 3 days (Femstat 3®). Gynazole-1® is a butoconazole topical preparation in a unique, prolonged, adherent preparation used as a single-dose agent.

Pharmacokinetics: About 5.5% is absorbed systemically via the vaginal walls.

Interactions: None reported.

Adverse events: Occasional sensitivity or chemical irritation may occur.

Precautions: Use only externally, avoid contact with eyes.

Pregnancy: Butoconazole is a category C drug; its safety for use during pregnancy has not been established.

Indications: Butoconazole is indicated for vulvovaginal candidiasis.

Tioconazole

Tioconazole (Vagistat-1®) is a synthetic, broad-spectrum imidazole.

Spectrum of activity: Tioconazole has in vitro activity against a broad range of fungi, including *C albicans*, non-*albicans Candida* species, and several dermatophytes. 7

Formulations: Tioconazole is available as a 6.5% vaginal cream.

Dosage: For vaginal candidiasis, insert one applicator intravaginally qhs as a single dose.

Pharmacokinetics: Negligible absorption.

Interactions: None reported.

Adverse events: Occasional sensitivity or chemical irritation may occur.

Precautions: Use only externally, avoid contact with eyes.

Pregnancy: Tioconazole is a category C agent; its safety for use during pregnancy has not been established.

Indications: Tioconazole is indicated for vulvovaginal candidiasis.

Terconazole

Terconazole (Terazol® 3, Terazol® 7) is a synthetic, broad-spectrum topical triazole.

Spectrum of activity: Terconazole has in vitro activity against a broad range of fungi, including *C albicans*, non-*albicans Candida* species, and several dermatophytes.

Formulations: Terconazole is available as a 0.4% vaginal cream in a 45-g tube or an 0.8% cream in a 20-g tube and as a 80-mg vaginal suppository.

Dosage: For vaginal candidiasis: 80-mg tablets; or insert 1 suppository (2.5 g) intravaginally qhs for 3 days, or insert 1 applicator (5 g) intravaginally qhs for 7 days; or apply 0.4% cream.

Pharmacokinetics: Only 5% to 16% of terconazole is absorbed. The drug is metabolized mainly in the liver, and 30% to 50% is excreted in the urine; 45% to 55% is excreted in the feces.

Interactions: None reported.

Adverse events: Occasional sensitivity or chemical irritation may occur.

Precautions: Use only externally, avoid contact with eyes.

Pregnancy: Terconazole is a category C agent; its safety for use during pregnancy has not been established.

Indications: Terconazole is indicated for vulvovaginal candidiasis.

Econazole Nitrate

Econazole nitrate (Spectazole®) is a synthetic, broad-spectrum topical imidazole.

Mechanism of action: Although econazole nitrate is an imidazole and exerts its effect on the inhibition of 14-α-lanosterol demethylase, electron microscopy studies have suggested that it also exerts a direct membrane-damaging effect on cytoplasmic organelles such as the mitochondria, nuclear membrane, and endoplasmic reticulum. In addition, econazole nitrate may suppress ATP production.

Spectrum of activity: Of all of the topical imidazoles, econazole has the broadest in vitro activity against a wide array of fungi, including *Candida* species, *Trichophyton rubrum*, *Trichophyton mentagrophytes*, *Epidermophyton floccosum*, *M canis*, and *Malassezia furfur*. In addition, it is highly active against *Aspergillus*, *Fusarium*, and *Penicillium* species.

Formulations: Econazole is available as a 1% water-soluble cream and a 1% ophthalmic solution.

Dosage: Gently rub onto affected area b.i.d. for 2 to 6 weeks.

Pharmacokinetics: Absorption through the skin is minimal.

Interactions: Corticosteroids can inhibit antifungal activity.

Adverse events: Burning, pruritus, and erythema are reported side effects.

Precautions: Use only externally, avoid contact with eyes.

Pregnancy: Econazole is a category C agent; its safety for use during pregnancy has not been established.

Indications: Econazole is indicated for cutaneous candidiasis, tinea pedis, tinea corporis, tinea cruris, pityriasis versicolor, and fungal keratitis.

Sulconazole Nitrate

Sulconazole (Exelderm®, Sulcosyn®) is a synthetic, broad-spectrum topical imidazole.

Spectrum of activity: Sulconazole has in vitro activity against *T rubrum*, *T mentagrophytes*, *E floccosum*, *M canis*, *M furfur*, *C albicans*, and *Aspergillus* species.

Formulations: Sulconazole is available as a 1% cream and solution.

Dosage: Gently rub onto affected area b.i.d. for 2 to 6 weeks.

Pharmacokinetics: Absorption through the skin is minimal.

Interactions: None reported.

Adverse events: Burning or pruritus is rare.

Precautions: Use only externally, avoid contact with eyes.

Pregnancy: Sulconazole is a category C agent; its safety for use during pregnancy has not been established.

Indications: Sulconazole is indicated for tinea pedis, tinea corporis, tinea cruris, pityriasis versicolor, and cutaneous candidiasis.

Oxiconazole Nitrate

Oxiconazole nitrate (Oxistat®) is a synthetic, broad-spectrum topical imidazole.

Spectrum of activity: Oxiconazole has in vitro activity against *T rubrum*, *T mentagrophytes*, *E floccosum*, *M canis*, *M furfur*, *A fumigatus*, *C neoformans*, *Rhizopus* species, and *C albicans*.

Formulations: Oxiconazole is available as a 1% cream and solution.

Dosage: Gently rub onto affected area b.i.d. for 2 to 6 weeks. May be used in pediatric patients.

Pharmacokinetics: Absorption through the skin is minimal; less than 0.3% of oxiconazole is excreted in the urine.

Interactions: None reported.

Adverse events: The incidence of burning, pruritus, and local irritation is <2%.

Precautions: Use only externally, avoid contact with eyes or vagina.

Pregnancy: Oxiconazole is a category B agent; it is usually safe, but benefits should outweigh the risks.

Indications: Oxiconazole is indicated for tinea pedis, tinea corporis, tinea cruris, and pityriasis versicolor.

Other Topical Azoles

Bifonazole

Bifonazole is a topical imidazole that has broad-spectrum in vitro activity against many pathogenic yeasts, dimorphic fungi, and filamentous fungi. It is weakly active against *Candida* and *Aspergillus* species.

Croconazole

Croconazole is a topical imidazole with broad-spectrum in vitro activity against a broad range of fungi, including *Aspergillus* species, *Penicillium* species, *T mentagrophytes*, *T rubrum*, *M canis*, *Microsporum gypseum*, *E floccosum*, *Candida* species, and *C neoformans*.

Uses: Croconazole's uses include the topical treatment of cutaneous candidiasis and dermatomycoses.

Fenticonazole

Fenticonazole is a topical imidazole with broad-spectrum in vitro activity against a wide array of fungi, including *T mentagrophytes*, *T rubrum*, *M canis*, *M gypseum*, and *E floccosum*. However, in the presence of acid pH, it also has in vitro activity against *Candida* species and *C neoformans*.

Mechanism of action: Although fenticonazole is an imidazole and exerts its effect on the inhibition of 14-α-lanosterol demethylase, electron microscopy studies have suggested that it also exerts a direct membrane-damaging effect on cytoplasmic organelles such as the mitochondria, nuclear membrane, and endoplasmic reticulum.

Uses: Fenticonazole is used to treat dermatomycosis and cutaneous and vaginal candidiasis.

Isoconazole

Isoconazole is a topical imidazole with broad-spectrum in vitro activity against a wide array of fungi, including *T mentagrophytes*, *T rubrum*, *M canis*, *E floccosum*, and numerous yeasts and fungi. One in vitro study found isoconazole to be more active than econazole, miconazole, and ketoconazole against several different *Candida* species.

Mechanism of action: Although isoconazole is an imidazole that affects 14-α-lanosterol demethylase activity, several investigators have suggested that it also damages the cellular membrane by lowering ATP concentrations.

Omoconazole

Omoconazole is a new topical imidazole with broad-spectrum in vitro activity against a wide array of fungi—comparable to the activity of clotrimazole, tioconazole, miconazole, econazole, and isoconazole—against *T mentagrophytes*, *T rubrum*, *M canis*, *E floccosum*, and numerous yeasts and fungi. It appears to be more active than those antifungals against *C neoformans*, *Pityrosporum* species, and *A fumigatus*.

Vibunazole

Vibunazole is a topical triazole with broad-spectrum, in vitro activity against many pathogenic fungi, including *Fusarium* species, *A fumigatus*, *C albicans*, and *C neoformans*. It can be used as oral or topical therapy.

Suggested Readings

Barriere SL: Pharmacology and pharmacokinetics of traditional systemic antifungal agents. *Pharmacotherapy* 1990;10:134S-140S.

Como J: Dismukes WE: Azole antifungal drugs. In: Dismukes WE, Pappas PG, Sobel JD, eds. *Clinical Mycology*, 1st ed. New York, NY, Oxford University Press, 2003, pp 64-87.

Ghannoum MA, Rice LB: Antifungal agents: mode of action, mechanism of resistance, and correlation of these mechanisms with bacterial resistance. *Clin Microbiol Rev* 1999;12:501-517.

Greenberg RN, Mullane K, van Berik JAH, et al: Posaconazole as salvage therapy for zygomycosis. *Antimicrob Agent Chemother* 2006;50:126-133.

Rex JH, Stevens DA: Antifungal agents. In: Mandell GL, Bennett JE, Dolin R, eds. *Principles and Practice of Infectious Diseases,* 6th ed. New York, NY, Churchill Livingstone, 2005, pp 502-513.

Chapter 8

Echinocandins (Pneumocandins)

Echinocandins are a new family of broad-spectrum synthetic lipopeptide antifungals that are derived from the fermentation broth of *Zalerion arboricola*. A subclass of echinocandins is called pneumocandins because of its activity against *Pneumocystis carinii* and *Candida* species. The echinocandins have become important front-line drugs of choice in the management of candidemia and systemic candidiasis, especially in patients who are hemodynamically unstable, in those who are moderately to severely septic from *Candida*, and in patients with known infection due to *Candida glabrata* and *Candida krusei*.

Mechanism of action: The mechanism of action of echinocandins is noncompetitive inhibition of the synthesis of the enzyme glucan synthase, which produces (1,3)β-D-glucan, an essential component of the cell wall of susceptible fungi. The destruction of the cell wall structure leads to osmotic instability and, ultimately, lysis of the fungal cell. (1,3)β-D-glucan is not present in mammalian cells.

Caspofungin

Caspofungin (Cancidas®) was the first of the new family of antifungal compounds that inhibit glucan synthase. It was approved by the US Food and Drug Administration (FDA) in January 2001. A semisynthetic, water-soluble pneumocandin, caspofungin acetate is derived from the fermentation products of *Glarea lozoyensis*.

Spectrum of activity: Caspofungin possesses in vitro activity against a broad range of fungi, including *Candida albicans*, many non-*albicans Candida* species (*C glabrata*, *C tropicalis*, *C krusei*, and *C lusitaniae*, with moderate activity against *C parapsilosis*), *Aspergillus fumigatus*, *Aspergillus flavus*, *Aspergillus terreus*, *Histoplasma capsulatum*, *Blastomyces dermatitidis*, *Coccidioides immitis*, and *Paracoccidioides brasiliensis*. Although there are limited data, caspofungin also appears to have limited activity against *Alternaria* species, *Curvularia lunata*, *Exophiala jeanselmei*, *Paecilomyces variotii*, *Scedosporium apiospermum*, and *Fonsecaea pedrosoi*.

Formulations: In adults, caspofungin is available in two dose strengths: a 70-mg IV solution and a 50-mg IV solution.

Dosage: Caspofungin should be administered in a 70-mg IV loading dose, followed by a daily 50-mg IV dose. Dosing in patients 3 months to 17 years of age is based on the patient's body surface area (BSA) as calculated by the Mosteller formula:

$$\text{BSA (m}^2\text{)} = \frac{\text{Height (cm) x weight (kg)}}{3600}$$

The loading dose in mg is BSA (m^2) x 70 mg/m^2. The maintenance dose is BSA (m^2) x 50 mg/m^2.

Pharmacokinetics: Oral absorption of caspofungin acetate is minimal. Distribution, instead of excretion or biotransformation, is the primary mechanism influencing plasma clearance. Plasma concentrations decline in a polyphasic manner, with a short initial-phase half-life, followed by a secondary phase (half-life of 9 to 11 hours). There is minimal excretion or metabolism of caspofungin during the first 30 hours after administration. There is minimal renal excretion of caspofungin and some hepatic metabolism by hydrolysis and N-acetylation. Less than 2% of the dose is excreted unchanged in the urine.

Interactions: Caspofungin reduces tacrolimus levels by approximately 20%. Cyclosporine increases caspofungin levels by approximately 35%; coadministration of both has led to transient increases in transaminases in about 10% of patients. In addition, coadministration of hepatic inducers and inducer/inhibitors (efavirenz [Sustiva®], nelfinavir [Viracept®], nevirapine [Viramune®], phenytoin, rifampin [Rifadin®, Rifadin®IV], dexamethasone, and carbamazepine (Carbatrol®, Tegretol®, Tegretol®-XR) may result in significant reductions in caspofungin levels. Caspofungin displays no antagonism or interaction with amphotericin B (Amphocin®, Fungizone®) or azoles. In vitro studies demonstrate additive/synergistic activity against many *Candida* and *Aspergillus* species when caspofungin is used with amphotericin B, fluconazole (Diflucan®), itraconazole (Sporanox®), or voriconazole (Vfend®).

Adverse events: Adverse events include phlebitis/thrombophlebitis (11% to 15%); increases in liver function test (aspartate aminotransferase, alanine aminotransferase, and alkaline phosphatase; 10% to 13%); and possible histamine-mediated symptoms, such as rash, facial edema, pruritus, and sensation of warmth (~3%).

Precautions: Patients who are receiving caspofungin and a hepatic inducer or inducer/inhibitor and are not responding to the usual dose of 50 mg/d should have the dosage increased to 70 mg/d. In patients with moderate hepatic insufficiency, after a loading dose of 70 mg, a daily dose of 35 mg should be used. Because there is minimal renal excretion, the daily dosage does not have to be modified for patients in renal failure. Caspofungin is not dialyzable; thus, supplementary dosing is not required after dialysis.

Pregnancy: Caspofungin is a category C drug. Its safety for use during pregnancy has not been established.

Indications: Caspofungin is now indicated in adult and pediatric patients (3 months and older). Caspofungin is indicated for the treatment of invasive aspergillosis in patients who are refractory to or intolerant of other antifungals, esophageal candidiasis, candidemia, and invasive candidiasis. A recently published clinical trial also indicated that caspofungin is as good as, if not superior to, amphotericin B in nonneutropenic patients with candidemia and disseminated candidiasis. In addition, caspofungin is also approved as empiric therapy for presumed fungal infections in febrile neutropenic patients.

Micafungin

Micafungin (Mycamine®), the second of the new family of antifungal compounds that inhibit glucan synthase, is a semisynthetic, water-soluble, cyclic hexapeptide echinocandin compound. It was approved by the FDA in May 2005.

Spectrum of activity: Micafungin possesses in vitro activity against a broad range of fungi, including *C albicans*, many non-*albicans Candida* species (*C glabrata, C tropicalis*, *C krusei*, and *C lusitaniae*, with moderate activity against *C parapsilosis*), *A fumigatus*, *A flavus*, *A niger*, *A terreus*, *H capsulatum*, *B dermatitidis*, and *C immitis*. Although there are limited data, micafungin also appears to have moderate activity against *Cladosporium trichoides*, *Exophiala dermatitidis*, *Exophiala spinifera*, and *F pedrosoi*.

Formulations: Micafungin is available in 50-mg and 100-mg vials.

Dosages: Micafungin was developed for parenteral use only. Micafungin should be administered at a dose of 150 mg/d for the treatment of esophageal candidiasis, at 50 mg/d when used for prophylaxis of *Candida* infections in hematopoietic stem cell transplant (HSCT) recipients, and at 100 mg/d for candidemia, acute disseminated candidiasis, *Candida* peritonitis, and *Candida* abscesses. A loading dose is not generally required. No dosing adjustments are required based on race, gender, or in patients with severe renal dysfunction or mild-to-moderate hepatic insufficiency.

Pharmacokinetics: Oral absorption of micafungin is minimal. Distribution, instead of excretion or biotransformation, is the primary mechanism influencing plasma clearance. Plasma concentrations decline in a biexponential pattern. The half-life ranges from 11.6-15.2 hours. Micafungin is highly (>99%) protein bound, independent of plasma levels. It is metabolized into at least six inert metabolites, via hydrolysis and acetylation, with minimal metabolism via the cytochrome P-450 enzyme system. There is minimal renal excretion, with less than 1% of the dose excreted unchanged. Fecal excretion is the major route of elimination.

Interactions: A total of 11 drug-drug interaction studies were conducted to evaluate the potential for interaction between micafungin and mycophenolate mofetil, cyclosporine, tacrolimus (Prograf®, Protopic®), prednisolone, sirolimus (Rapamune®), nifedipine (Adalat® CC), fluconazole, ritonavir, and rifampin. In these studies, no interaction that altered the pharmacokinetics of micafungin was observed. 8
Sirolimus AUC was increased by 21% with no effect on C_{max} in the presence of steady-state micafungin compared with sirolimus alone. Nifedipine AUC and C_{max} were increased by 18% and 42%, respectively, in the presence of steady-state micafungin compared with nifedipine alone. Patients receiving sirolimus or nifedipine in combination with micafungin should be monitored for sirolimus or nifedipine toxicity and sirolimus or nifedipine dosage should be reduced if necessary.

Adverse events: Clinical trials with micafungin have reported few adverse events. The more common include nausea, vomiting, and headaches (2.4% to 2.8%); increase in liver function tests, aspartate aminotransferase, alanine aminotransferase, and alkaline phosphatase (2.0% to 2.7%); and rare histamine-mediated symptoms, such as pruritus, rash, and flushing (<2%).

Precautions: Because there is minimal renal excretion, the daily dosage does not have to be modified for patients in renal failure. Micafungin is not dialyzable; thus, supplementary dosing is not required after dialysis.

Pregnancy: Micafungin is a category C drug. Its safety for use during pregnancy has not been established.

Indications: Micafungin is indicated for the treatment of patients with esophageal candidiasis, for prophylaxis of

Candida infections in patients undergoing hematopoietic stem cell transplantation, and for the treatment of candidemia, acute disseminated candidiasis, *Candida* peritonitis, and *Candida* abscesses. In addition, a phase III clinical trial also indicated that micafungin is as good as AmBisome® in patients with candidemia and invasive candidiasis.

Anidulafungin

Anidulafungin (Eraxis™) is the third in the family of new antifungal compounds that inhibit glucan synthase. It is a semisynthetic echinocandin that was approved by the FDA in February 2006.

Spectrum of activity: Anidulafungin possesses in vitro activity against a broad range of fungi, including *C albicans*, many non-*albicans Candida* species (*C glabrata*, *C tropicalis*, *C krusei*, and *C lusitaniae*, with moderate activity against *C parapsilosis*). It also displays activity against *A fumigatus, A flavus, A terreus, Histoplasma capsulatum, Blastomyces dermatitidis, Coccidioides immitis*, and *Paracoccidioides braziliensis*. Although there are limited data, anidulafungin also appears to have some activity against *Alternaria* species, *Curvularia lunata, Exophiala jeanselmei, Paecilomyces variotii, Scedosporium apiospermum*, and *Fonsecaea pedrosoi*.

Formulations: Anidulafungin is supplied in 50-mg and 100-mg vials for IV administration.

Dosage: Anidulafungin should be administered at a dose of 200 mg loading dose, followed by 100 mg daily thereafter for candidemia and deep tissue candidiasis. In esophageal candidiasis, anidulafungin is administered at 100 mg loading dose, followed by 50 mg daily thereafter.

Pharmacokinetics: Oral absorption of anidulafungin is minimal. Anidulafungin is unique even among other echinocandins, as it slowly degrades in human plasma, undergoing a process of biotransformation rather than being metabolized. As with caspofungin and micafungin, the compound is only administered intravenously. An initial loading dose of twice the daily dose achieves a level near steady state within 24 h after the first dose. In vitro studies have shown that anidulafungin is protein bound (~96%) to human plasma.

The echinocandins consist of an amphophilic hexapeptide ring with a lipid side that in anidulafungin is an alkoxytriphenyl chain. More than 90% of anidulafungin undergoes a slow chemical degradation in the blood and does not involve the hepatic cytochrome CYP-450 system. Initially, it is degraded into an open-ringed product that is then degraded by nonspecific peptidases into inactive compounds. As observed in both human and animal pharmacokinetic studies, the half-life of anidulafungin is approximately 24 h, whereas the half-life of the degradation products is approximately 4 days. Minimal drug or drug degradation products are found in the urine. Most anidulafungin degradation products pass into the feces via the biliary tree. The significance of this high degree of degradation instead of metabolism is important for anidulafungin's minimal drug-drug interaction profile.

Interactions: Anidulafungin is not metabolized by the human cychrome P-450 and does not affect the activities of clinically important human CYP (1A2, 2C9, 2D6, 3A4). No clinically relevant drug-drug interactions were observed with drugs likely to be co-administered with anidulafungin. Drug interaction studies with cyclosporine, voriconazole, tacrolimus, AmBisome®, and rifampin were conducted. In these studies, no interactions altering pharmacokinetics were observed.

Adverse events: Anidulafungin has reported few adverse events. The more common include nausea, vomiting, diarrhea, dyspepsia (0.5% to 3.9%), elevations in liver function test (ALT, AST, alkaline phosphatase 1% to 2%), rash, and hypokalemia (<3%). As with other echinocandins, possible histamine-mediated reactions have been reported including rash, urticaria, flushing, pruritus, and hypotension.

Precautions: Because there is minimal renal excretion, the daily dosage does not have to be modified for patients in renal failure. Anidulafungin is not dialyzable, thus supplementary dosing is not required after dialysis.

Pregnancy: Anidulafungin is a category C drug. Its safety for use during pregnancy has not been established.

Indications: Anidulafungin is indicated as treatment for esophageal candidiasis, candidemia, and other *Candida* infections, including peritonitis and intra-abdominal absesses.

Suggested Readings

Deresinski SC, Stevens DA: Caspofungin. *Clin Infect Dis* 2003;36: 1445-1457.

DiDomenico B: Novel antifungal drugs. *Curr Opin Microbiol* 1999; 2:509-515.

Ghannoum MA, Rice LB: Antifungal agents: mode of action, mechanism of resistance, and correlation of these mechanisms with bacterial resistance. *Clin Microbiol Rev* 1999;12:501-517.

Groll AH, Walser TJ: Cell wall synthesis inhibitors: echinocandins and nikkomycins. In: Dismukes WE, Pappas PG, Sobel JD, eds. *Clinical Mycology*, 1st ed. New York, NY, Oxford University Press, 2003, pp 88-103.

Hossain MA, Reyes GH, Ghannoum MA: Newer antifungal agents and treatment strategies. *Rev Med Microbiol* 2001;12(suppl 1): S3-S12.

Mora-Durate J, Betts R, Rotstein C, et al: Comparison of caspofungin and amphotericin B for invasive candidiasis. *N Engl J Med* 2002; 347:2020-2029.

Rex JH, Stevens DA: Systemic antifungal agents. In: Mandell GL, Bennett JE, Dolin R, eds. *Principles and Practice of Infectious Diseases*, 6th ed. New York, NY Churchill Livingstone, 2005, pp 502-513.

van Burik JH, Ratanatharathorn V, Stepan DE, et al: micafungin versus fluconazole for prophylaxis against invasive fungal infections during neutropenia in patients undergoing hematopoietic stem cell transplantation. *Clin Infect Dis* 2004;39:1407-1416.

Vazquez JA: Anidulafungin: a novel echinocandin. *Therapy* 2006; 3:39-54.

Vazquez JA: Anidulafungin: a new echinocandin with a novel profile. *Clin Ther* 2005;27:657-653.

Chapter 9

Allylamines

The allylamines are a family of synthetic broad-spectrum antifungals that are predominantly used for skin and nail infections.

Mechanism of action: Allylamines inhibit ergosterol synthesis via inhibition of squalene epoxidase. This enzyme is part of the fungal sterol synthesis pathway that generates the sterols required by fungal cell membranes, and its inhibition results in the death of the fungal cell. The allylamines exhibit fungicidal activity against a broad group of fungi, including dermatophytes, molds, and some yeasts, but they are fungistatic against *Candida* species.

Terbinafine

Terbinafine (Lamisil®) is a synthetic allylamine derivative with broad-spectrum antifungal activity.

Spectrum of activity: Terbinafine has in vitro activity against *Trichophyton rubrum, Trichophyton mentagrophytes, Trichophyton verrucosum, Microsporum canis, Microsporum gypseum, Microsporum nanum, Candida* species, *Epidermophyton floccosum, Scopulariopsis brevicaulis, Aspergillus* species, *Sporothrix schenckii, Penicillium marneffei, Cryptococcus neoformans,* and *Trichosporon* and *Blastoschizomyces* species.

Formulations: Terbinafine is available in 250-mg tablets and 1% cream and solution.

Dosage: The following dosages are used in oral therapy: fingernail onychomycosis, 250 mg/d PO for 6 weeks, not to exceed 12 weeks; toenail infections, 250 mg/d PO for 12 weeks. Pediatric dosages are weight based: <20 kg, 67.5 mg/d PO; 20 to 40 kg, 125 mg/d PO; >40 kg, 250 mg/d PO. The duration should be as in adults. Topical preparations should be applied to the affected area twice daily for 1 to 4 weeks.

Pharmacokinetics: After oral administration, terbinafine is well absorbed, with a bioavailability of >75%. It is highly lipophilic and tends to accumulate in the skin, nails, and tissues. Its terminal half-life is approximately 200 to 400 hours. Terbinafine is extensively metabolized in the liver, and about 70% of the dose is excreted in the urine.

Interactions: Terbinafine increases clearance of cyclosporine by 15%. Terbinafine clearance is increased 100% by rifampin and decreased 33% by cimetidine.

Adverse events: The most frequently reported effects are gastrointestinal, including diarrhea, dyspepsia, and abdominal pain. Rashes, urticaria, pruritus, liver function test elevations, taste disturbances, and rare ocular opacities have been reported. Rare cases of symptomatic cholestasis have also been reported.

Precautions: Terbinafine is not recommended in patients with a creatinine clearance <50 mL/min and should be used with caution in patients with impaired hepatic function. Patients on long-term therapy should have ophthalmologic evaluations. Liver function tests are recommended in patients administered terbinafine for more than 6 weeks. Hematologic toxicity is occasionally seen with neutropenia and anemias. A complete blood count with differential is recommended every 6 weeks.

Pregnancy: Terbinafine is a category B drug. It is usually safe, but the benefits should outweigh the risks.

Uses: Oral therapy is used for onychomycosis; topical therapy is used for tinea corporis, tinea cruris, tinea pedis, and pityriasis versicolor.

Suggested Reading

Ghannoum MA, Rice LB: Antifungal agents: mode of action, mechanism of resistance, and correlation of these mechanisms with bacterial resistance. *Clin Microbiol Rev* 1999;12:501-517.

Pappas GP: Terbinafine. In: Dismukes WE, Pappas PG, Sobel JD, eds. *Clinical Mycology*. 1st ed. New York, NY, Oxford University Press, 2003, pp 104-110.

Rex JH, Stevens DA: Systemic antifungal agents. In: Mandell GL, Bennett JE, Dolin R, eds. *Principles and Practice of Infectious Diseases*. 6th ed. New York, NY Churchill Livingstone, 2005, pp 502-515.

Chapter **10**

Antifungal Resistance

Infections with strains of yeast that are resistant or less susceptible to antifungal agents have recently been described in HIV-negative populations. There are many reports of severe infection with *Candida krusei* or *Candida glabrata* with widespread in vitro antifungal resistance. Even *Candida* species resistant to amphotericin B (Amphocin®, Fungizone®), rare in the past, have recently been reported.

The role of fungi in the severely immunocompromised host has expanded greatly since the AIDS epidemic. This epidemic, in conjunction with the release of safe and effective antifungals, has produced a new era in medical mycology: the era of antifungal resistance. Clinicians need to be aware of this problem, use antifungals judiciously, and be vigilant for the development of resistance.

Currently, the problem of antifungal resistance seems to be limited to patients with severely compromised immune function, primarily patients with AIDS. Much still needs to be learned about the epidemiology, pathogenesis, management, and prevention of resistant fungal infections.

Azole antifungal resistance was virtually nonexistent before the emergence of HIV disease. Although imidazole-resistant strains have been described since 1978, the lack of a standardized, reliable in vitro susceptibility method makes the older literature difficult to interpret. Numerous reports describing antifungal-refractory mucosal candidiasis have been published over the past 10 years. More than 50 reports describing antifungal resistance in the HIV-positive patient have been published in the world literature in the past 12 years. Refractory candidiasis has emerged as an important opportunistic disease that affects patients with advanced HIV infection. Subsequently, fungal infections have become an important cause of morbidity and mortality in patients with HIV/AIDS.

The overall estimated frequency of azole resistance is still unknown, but it is approximated to be 4% to 6% for *Candida albicans* isolates recovered from patients with AIDS. The frequency of resistance to other azole compounds, such as clotrimazole (Mycelex®, Lotrimin®), itraconazole (Sporanox®), and ketoconazole (Nizoral®), is unknown but speculated to be slightly lower.

Classification of Resistance

Antifungal resistance can be divided into two levels: clinical and cellular (in vitro). Clinical resistance is not necessarily caused by a failure of the antifungal or associated with reduced in vitro susceptibility. Clinical failure is usually a result of low levels of the drug in serum and/or tissues, which can be caused by poor patient adherence, drug-drug interactions that decrease antifungal levels, or, in the patient with AIDS, severe immunosuppression. If the host immune system is severely impaired or nonfunctional, even high doses of fungicidal agents will not eradicate the fungal infection.

Cellular (in vitro) resistance is independent of the host and involves strains that are less responsive to antifungals at the standard doses. Most reports of azole resistance describe fluconazole (Diflucan®) resistance in patients with advanced HIV infection. Recently, Maenza et al identified several key risk factors for the development of fluconazole-resistant mucocutaneous candidal disease. These risk factors include more episodes of oropharyngeal candidiasis (OPC) than in controls (3.1 episodes vs 1.8 episodes), lower median $CD4^+$ lymphocyte cell count (11 cells/mm^3 vs 71 cells/mm^3), greater median duration of prior antifungal therapy (419 days vs 118 days), and systemic azole use (272 days vs 14 days). When Maenza et al paired the cases with two sets of controls matched by CD4$^+$ cell count, resistant cases continued to show a greater median exposure time to azoles (272 days vs 88 days) as a significant risk factor for fluconazole-resistant OPC.

There are several known cellular mechanisms of resistance. *Primary* (intrinsic) *resistance* is demonstrated by organisms that are naturally resistant to an antifungal (eg, *Aspergillus terreus* is intrinsically resistant to amphotericin B). The best example of this type of resistance has been described in *C krusei,* which is accepted to be intrinsically resistant to fluconazole and is frequently resistant to other azoles, such as itraconazole, ketoconazole, and clotrimazole. Other examples of primary resistance include replacement of the original isolate by a more resistant species or by a more resistant strain of the same species, genetic alterations in the original strain that result in a more resistant strain, and transient gene expression that renders the fungal cell temporarily resistant. The term *secondary* (acquired) *resistance* is used when an initially susceptible isolate becomes resistant to an antifungal agent. This form of resistance was rare in the past, but it is now repeatedly encountered, predominantly in HIV-positive patients, and reported in the literature.

The methodology used to perform in vitro susceptibility studies for *Candida* species is now standardized and uniform, but it has some limitations.

Susceptibility Testing and Definition of Resistance

A clear definition of resistance is important to evaluating resistance patterns. Efforts to develop standardized, reproducible, and clinically relevant testing methods have resulted in the development of the CLSI NCCLS M27-A methodology for susceptibility testing of yeasts. Data-driven breakpoints are available for testing the susceptibility of

Table 10-1: Interpretive Breakpoints for *Candida* Species

Drug	Minimum Inhibitory Concentration (μg/mL) Susceptible	Susceptible–dose dependent	Resistant
Fluconazole (Diflucan®)	≤8	16-32	>32
Itraconazole (Sporanox®)	≤0.125	0.25-0.5	>0.5
Flucytosine (Ancobon®)	<4	8-16	>16

Candida species to fluconazole, itraconazole, and flucytosine (Ancobon®) (Table 10-1). Reliable breakpoints are not yet available for amphotericin B.

Mechanisms of Resistance and Clinical Relevance

The mechanisms of resistance to antifungals, including amphotericin B, are still poorly understood because antifungal resistance has only recently become a problem. Alterations in the sterol concentrations of the plasma membranes and changes in the lipid composition of the cell membrane have been reported. An observed alteration in plasma membrane sterol is postulated to be the cause of resistance in one amphotericin B cross-resistant *C albicans* isolate.

Amphotericin B Resistance

We recovered a series of *Candida guilliermondii* isolates that demonstrated in vivo conversion of amphotericin B susceptibility to amphotericin B resistance over a 4-week period while the patient was on high-dose amphotericin B and flucytosine. However, few studies have evaluated the molecular mechanisms of resistance in yeasts or fungi, and the clinical relevance of antifungal resistance and antifungal tolerance has been infrequently demonstrated. In one study, Powderly et al observed an almost 100% mortality rate in patients infected with strains of yeast that were tolerant of or resistant to amphotericin B (minimum inhibitory concentration [MIC] of amphotericin B , >0.8 μg/mL). Among patients infected with strains of yeast sensitive to amphotericin B (MIC of amphotericin B <0.8 μg/mL), the mortality rate was 50%. Recently, there have been several reports of amphotericin B resistance in *C albicans* isolates from patients without HIV. There have also been several reports of *Cryptococcus neoformans* isolates resistant to amphotericin B .

Flucytosine Resistance

Flucytosine resistance has been extensively described. Primary resistance rates in *Candida* species vary from 5% to 50%, depending on the species and the technique used to perform the susceptibility studies. Overall, *Candida tropicalis, C krusei,* and *Candida parapsilosis* have greater primary resistance rates than do *C albicans* and *C glabrata.* Rates of primary resistance to flucytosine vary widely for other fungal organisms. *Cryptococcus* species have an intrinsic resistance rate of 1% to 4 %, whereas most *Aspergillus* species are resistant to flucytosine, as are the dimorphic fungi, *Histoplasmosis capsulatum, Coccidioides immitis, Sporothrix schenckii,* and *Blastomyces dermatitidis.*

The development of secondary resistance to flucytosine in *Candida* species is common and has been well documented. The risk of resistance seems to be directly proportional to several coexisting factors, including fungal burden, frequency of mutation resulting in secondary resistance in a particular *Candida* strain, low flucytosine concentrations (<25 μg/mL) in tissue or serum, use of flucytosine monotherapy, presence of *Candida* in the urinary tract, and degree of immunosuppression. It has been reported that more than 60% of *Candida* isolates recovered from patients receiving flucytosine as monotherapy have developed resistance during therapy. In addition, in vitro resistance can be easily induced in *Candida* and *Cryptococcus* species in the laboratory when the organisms are grown in low concentrations of flucytosine on liquid or solid media.

There are four well-known major mechanisms of flucytosine resistance: (1) deficiency in cytosine permease, (2) deficiency in cytosine deaminase, (3) deficiency in UMP pyrophosphorylase, and (4) loss of feedback regulation leading to increased de novo synthesis of pyrimidines. There is no evidence of cross-resistance with different families of antifungals.

It is strongly recommended that the use of flucytosine be limited to adjunctive or combination therapy and that flucytosine not be used as monotherapy. It is also advisable to maintain serum drug levels of more than 25 μg/mL, and preferably between 25 and 50 μg/mL, to deter the development of secondary resistance in vivo.

Azole Resistance

There are several known molecular mechanisms of resistance to the azole class of antifungals. In *Candida* species, they include (1) changes in the sterol components of the plasma membrane, preventing antifungals from entering the cell; (2) genetic changes in the *ERG11* gene (14α-LDM, lanosterol demethylase), including point mutations in *ERG11,* which make the enzyme less susceptible to the azole; enzyme overexpression of 14-LDM, which leads to increased production of the azole target molecule; and gene amplification of 14-LDM, which leads to overexpression; (3) alterations in other enzymes in the ergosterol biosynthetic pathway, such as $\Delta^{5\text{-}6}$-sterol desaturase; and (4) drug efflux mechanisms. Low levels of active efflux systems are naturally present in all yeast cells.

Two low-level active efflux systems, the ATP-binding cassette (ABC) transporters and the major facilitators, pump out a small amount of all antifungal agents. The ABC transporters are associated with drug resistance in a wide variety of organisms. The genes *CDR1* and *CDR2* encode several components of the ABC transporters, including a transmembrane pore composed of several segments and two ATP-binding cassettes that are situated on the cytosolic side of the membrane and provide metabolic energy for the pump. To date, at least 13 ABC transporter efflux pumps have been described in *C albicans*. The major facilitators are primarily composed of 12 to 14 transmembrane segments and use the proton motive force of the membrane as a source of energy. To date, the only major facilitator gene that has been cloned in *Candida* is *MDR1*. Several studies have suggested that *MDR1* overexpression correlates with azole resistance in clinical isolates.

The problem of azole resistance is complicated by primary and secondary resistance and by patients' HIV status. In the non-HIV/AIDS setting, primary azole resistance tends to be associated with nosocomial colonization and infection. Several recent reports describe an increase in the isolation of non-*albicans Candida* species, specifically *C krusei* and *C glabrata*. *Candida krusei* is well known for its intrinsic resistance to fluconazole and is generally a nosocomially acquired, institution-specific pathogen. It is also frequently resistant or less susceptible to other antifungals such as ketoconazole, clotrimazole, miconazole (Micatin®, Monistat®), and amphotericin B. Of greater significance is *C glabrata,* which is emerging as one of the most common clinical isolates recovered from blood cultures. Overall, *C glabrata* tends to have higher MICs and thus is less susceptible to all antifungals, including amphotericin B. Secondary resistance in the non-HIV setting is still extremely uncommon.

The first case of azole resistance was described in 1978 in a child with a miconazole-resistant *Candida* urinary tract infection. Before the AIDS epidemic and the release and use of fluconazole, most cases of documented antifungal resistance were described in patients who had chronic mucocutaneous candidiasis and were on long-term suppressive therapy with ketoconazole. There are relatively few recent case reports of fluconazole-resistant *C albicans* producing disease in HIV-negative patients. In a recent report, Goff et al described the isolation of 37 strains of fluconazole-resistant *C albicans* recovered from patients at a university medical center. The patients had never received fluconazole. Twenty of the 37 isolates were recovered from patients who did not have HIV. Genotyping of the isolates was not performed, but fluconazole-resistant isolates from patients with AIDS were recovered in the same medical center, and the patients without HIV may have acquired the yeast from the environment.

One of the first cases of azole resistance in a patient with AIDS was described in 1986. Tavitian et al described six patients with HIV infection and esophageal candidiasis managed with standard doses of oral ketoconazole. On the follow-up visit, all six patients had recurrent esophageal disease. *Candida albicans* isolates recovered from the esophagi of two patients were resistant to ketoconazole in vitro.

Sobel and Vazquez have described the first case of outpatient-acquired fluconazole-resistant vaginal candidiasis in an HIV-negative host. This patient had been taking several over-the-counter antifungals as well as oral fluconazole for some time before she was seen in the clinic for a refractory vaginal infection. Her isolate, unlike other isolates described in the literature, had a high degree of cross-resistance to ketoconazole, clotrimazole, and itraconazole. However, it was still susceptible to miconazole, flucytosine, and amphotericin B. The high degree of cross-resistance may have been produced by the patient's use of over-the-counter azole antifungal preparations. This type of high-level azole cross-resistance has been previously described only in patients with end-stage or advanced AIDS who have had multiple episodes of mucocutaneous candidiasis and have been prescribed numerous courses of topical and systemic antifungals.

In 1995, Nguyen et al reported several cases of fluconazole-resistant *C parapsilosis* fungemia in hospitalized patients who were immunocompromised but not HIV positive.

Most cases of azole resistance described in the literature involve fluconazole in AIDS patients. The high prevalence of OPC and esophageal candidiasis in these severely compromised patients and the long-term use of fluconazole for acute treatment or prophylaxis of fungal infections have led to numerous reports of clinical failure and in vitro resistance to fluconazole in these patients.

Several molecular epidemiologic studies have been performed to further clarify the pathogenesis and evolution of fluconazole-resistant *Candida* infections. Many of these studies have demonstrated that in most cases of resistance, the same strain of yeast is present before and after the development of resistance. This generally indicates an in vivo conversion of one strain of *Candida* into a resistant phenotype. One study evaluated isolates from a husband and wife with fluconazole-resistant OPC. Using genotyping techniques, the authors demonstrated genetic similarity, suggesting that the resistant isolates were transmitted between partners.

Of great concern is the recent discovery of azole cross-resistance during antifungal therapy in AIDS patients with fluconazole-refractory OPC. In one study, 45 isolates from 41 patients who failed at least 400 mg/d of fluconazole underwent in vitro susceptibility testing. Twenty-seven *C albicans* isolates had MICs >20 µg/mL to fluconazole, 41% were cross-resistant to clotrimazole, and 11% were cross-resistant to itraconazole and ketoconazole. Of 14 fluconazole-resistant *C glabrata* isolates recovered from the same population, 86% were cross-resistant to clotrimazole, 57% were cross-resistant to ketoconazole, and 64% were cross-resistant to itraconazole.

Azole cross-resistance is of greatest concern in patients with AIDS, especially those with severe depletion of $CD4^+$ cells and associated high viral burdens, who frequently acquire multiple fungal infections. These patients generally require prolonged repeat courses of antifungals and have recurring fungal infections. However, in vitro azole resistance does not explain all therapeutic failures. Further work is required to explain failure of treatment despite adequate serum concentrations of antifungals and in vitro susceptibility of the isolates.

Clinical failure in a patient with advanced AIDS seems to be a harbinger of end-stage AIDS and severe immunosuppression. It is generally limited to AIDS patients who have $CD4^+$ cell counts below 50 cells/mm^3 and who have had several episodes of mucosal candidiasis and repeat courses of systemic antifungals. However, these patients are frequently hospitalized, and investigators have proven that *Candida* isolates can be transmitted between patients, hospital personnel, and the environment. Resistant *Candida* strains could therefore become an important cause of nosocomial fungal infections in patients without HIV. Recalcitrant/resistant mucosal candidiasis is not a life-threatening disease, but it seems to be associated with a shortened life expectancy and high morbidity and mortality in affected patients. These patients frequently suffer from continual malnutrition, dehydration, and wasting because they cannot maintain adequate oral intake. Much still needs to be learned about the epidemiology, pathogenesis, management, and prevention of resistant fungal infections.

Echinocandin Resistance

Echinocandins are a relatively new class of synthetic antifungal that act by noncompetitive inhibition of the synthesis of (1,3)-β-D-glucan synthase. Until now, resistance to echinocandin has been rare.

Because echinocandins are a recent addition to the antifungal armamentarium, few cases of clinical resistance have been reported. Hernandez et al reported on a *C albicans* strain recovered from a patient with AIDS and esophageal candidiasis. The *C albicans* displayed resistance to caspofungin. In a separate case, Moudgal et al reported a case of prosthetic valve endocarditis caused by *C parapsilosis*. The *C parapsilosis* developed in vivo resistance to caspofungin (Cancidas®), micafungin (Mycamine®), fluconazole, and voriconazole (Vfend®). It did remain susceptible to amphotericin B and anidulafungin (Eraxis™). Echinocandin resistance appears to be due, in part, to mutations in the FKS genes, FKS1 and FKS2, encoding (1,3)-β-D-glucan synthase. The exact mechanisms for cross-echinocandin resistance is still unknown.

Management of Resistant Mucocutaneous Candidiasis

Successful management of any disease requires a full understanding of its epidemiology, etiology, and pathogenesis and the actions and effects of available therapy. Management of antifungal-resistant mucocutaneous candidiasis is frequently unsatisfactory, and response is short lived, with periodic and rapid recurrence. Recent advances in understanding the epidemiology, the host, the organism, and the response to therapy have greatly altered the way clinicians manage acute candidiasis and advise primary prophylaxis and secondary prophylaxis. Preventing dangerous sequelae such as refractory candidiasis, wasting syndrome, and subsequent death has emerged as a major challenge.

Recently, AIDS Clinical Trial Group Study 819, a multicenter, prospective study of the risk factors, natural history, and outcome of fluconazole-refractory mucosal candidiasis, was completed. The investigators found an overall

Table 10-2: Alternative Therapy for the Management of Antifungal-refractory Mucosal Candidiasis in Patients with AIDS*

Antifungals

- High-dose fluconazole (Diflucan®) (800-1600 mg/d)
- Fluconazole oral suspension
- Itraconazole (Sporanox®) oral solution
- Posaconazole (Noxafil®)
- Amphotericin B oral solution
- Parenteral amphotericin B
- Liposomal formulations of amphotericin B
- Voriconazole (Vfend®)
- Caspofungin acetate (Cancidas®)
- Anidulafungin (Eraxis™)
- Micafungin (Mycamine®)

Combination Therapy

- Amphotericin B + flucytosine (Ancobon®)
- Amphotericin B + fluconazole
- Fluconazole + flucytosine
- rhuGM-CSF + fluconazole
- Fluconazole + terbinafine (Lamisil®)
- Fluconazole + caspofungin
- Voriconazole + anidulafungin

Investigational Antifungal Agents

- *Melaleuca* oral solution

*Many of the alternative therapies are not approved by the US Food and Drug Administration and are not supported by adequate clinical trials. rhuGM-CSF = recombinant human granulocyte-macrophage colony-stimulating factor.

fluconazole resistance risk of 4.3% over a 2-year period. In a multivariate analysis, the use of and trimethoprim/sulfamethoxazole (TMP/SMX) (Bactrim™, Septra®) and fluconazole was significantly associated with the development of fluconazole-refractory mucosal candidiasis. After the development of refractory candidiasis, the median survival of HIV-infected patients was 32.6 weeks. Thus, the development of refractory disease was an indicator of poor prognosis in HIV-positive patients. Although mucocutaneous candidiasis does not directly cause death, clinical antifungal failure is probably a comorbidity factor in the rapid demise of these patients. On the other hand, clinical failure may be a marker of severe immunosuppression and advanced dysfunction of the immune system.

In some patients, refractory candidiasis may respond to an increased dose of fluconazole (Table 10-2). For example, if the patient is failing therapy with fluconazole 200 mg/d, a dosage increase to 400 mg/d will frequently produce a temporary clinical response. However, the disease usually recurs once patients have reached this stage. Clinical and in vitro resistance to clotrimazole is frequent when patients fail to respond to fluconazole. Fluconazole suspension has proven to be beneficial in some patients with fluconazole-refractory OPC. Increased salivary levels obtained with the swish-and-swallow technique may account for this improvement.

Several studies evaluating itraconazole oral solution have demonstrated promising results in patients with AIDS who had failed fluconazole 200 mg/d. Clinical cure or improvement occurred in 55% to 70% of patients. Mycologic cure rates were low (<30%), and relapses following treatment cessation were rapid, usually within 14 days. Therefore, patients at this level who respond to an antifungal should be kept on a maintenance regimen until their immune function has been restored.

Amphotericin B oral suspension is a possible therapeutic option in patients with azole-refractory mucosal candidiasis.

In several small studies, clinical improvement rates varied from 50% to 75%, but as with all such patients, the relapse rate was high, and relapse occurred within 4 weeks of stopping therapy.

Posaconazole is now FDA approved for the treatment of oropharyngeal candidiasis that is refractory to itraconazole and/or fluconazole. In a recent open-label study, posaconazole 400 mg PO b.i.d. was effective in eradicating 86% of fluconazole or itraconazole refractory oropharyngeal or esophageal candidiasis in HIV/AIDS patients.

In a separate open-labeled clinical trial, anidulafungin IV at 50 mg/d was used to treat 19 patients with azole refractory mucosal candidiasis. At the end of therapy (21 days), clinical success was observed in 92% of patients.

Parenteral amphotericin B at dosages of 0.4 to 0.6 mg/kg/d may be required to achieve response in patients with severe disease. After the therapeutic response is obtained, it is essential to continue suppressive amphotericin B therapy in an attempt to increase disease-free intervals.

Unfortunately, not all patients respond to amphotericin B. In a small subpopulation of patients, even dosages of 1 mg/kg/d may not ameliorate signs and symptoms of mucocutaneous candidiasis. These patients generally have advanced HIV disease and, ultimately, high viral burdens and uncontrolled HIV infection. Several clinical trials are evaluating liposomal preparations of amphotericin B for refractory OPC. These preparations may prove useful in patients who cannot tolerate amphotericin B because of its nephrotoxicity or bone marrow suppression.

Future Therapeutic Strategy

Several new antifungal compounds are in clinical trials and appear to be encouraging. Two extended-spectrum triazoles, voriconazole and posaconazole, have excellent in vitro activity against fluconazole-resistant isolates. The echinocandins caspofungin and micafungin also have excellent antifungal activity. Promising in vitro results have been obtained against many *Candida* species, including fluconazole-resistant *C albicans, C glabrata,* and *C krusei.*

The significance of the dysfunctional immune system in patients with AIDS and refractory fungal infections should not be underestimated. Highly active antiretroviral therapy (HAART) could lower HIV viral loads, increase $CD4^+$ cell counts, and improve the immune function of a patient with advanced HIV infection, and it may help resolve refractory fungal infections. Treatment with HAART alone, without antifungals, has eradicated antifungal-refractory OPC in patients with advanced HIV infection.

The classic management of infection in the compromised host has always depended on antimicrobial agents, without accounting for host deficiencies. Several cytokines developed and produced by recombinant technology show promise in assisting the host response to fungal infection. There have been several reports of use of recombinant human granulocyte-macrophage colony stimulating factor (rhuGM-CSF) in patients with OPC or esophageal candidiasis refractory to fluconazole and amphotericin B . Although no large studies have been published, the few case reports describe good response rates with rhuGM-CSF in patients with advanced HIV infection and refractory mucosal candidiasis. Further studies evaluating these new cytokines are warranted.

Alternative therapeutic modalities using organic substances are also being administered empirically to combat refractory mucosal candidiasis. One of these substances is *Melaleuca alternifolia (*Australian tea tree) oil that has been formulated into an oral solution. A small, single-center pilot study using the solution in 14 patients with AIDS and fluconazole-refractory OPC was recently completed. The results seem to indicate relatively good efficacy in these difficult-to-treat patients, with clinical response in 10 of 12 patients after 4 weeks. However, larger comparative studies are necessary to evaluate the role of this agent in refractory candidiasis.

Suggested Readings

Ghannoum MA, Rice LB: Antifungal agents: mode of action, mechanism of resistance, and correlation of these mechanisms with bacterial resistance. *Clin Microbiol Rev* 1999;12:501-517.

Hernandez S, Lopez-Ribot JL, Najron LK, et al: Caspofungin resistance in *Candida albicans*: correlating clinical outcome with laboratory susceptibility testing of three isogenic isolates serially obtained from a patient with progressive *Candida esophagitis*. *Antimicrob Agents Chemother* 2004;48:1382-1383.

Moudgal V, Little T, Boikov D, et al: Multiechinocandin and multiazole-resistant *Candida parapsilosis* isolates serially obtained during therapy for prosthetic valve endocarditis. *Antimicrob Agent Chemother* 2005;49:767-769.

Sanglard D: Resistance to antifungal drugs. In: Dismukes WE, Pappas PG, Sobel JD, eds. *Clinical Mycology.* 1st ed. New York, NY, Oxford University Press, 2003, pp 111-124.

Vazquez JA: Therapeutic options for the management of oropharyngeal and esophageal candidiasis in HIV/AIDS patients. *HIV Clin Trials* 2000;1:47-59.

Vazquez JA, Sobel JD: Epidemiologic overview of resistance to oral antifungal agents in the immunocompromised host. *Excerpta Med Abstr J* Amsterdam, Elsevier Science BV, 1997, pp 1-11.

White TC, Marr KA, Bowden RA: Clinical, cellular, and molecular factors that contribute to antifungal drug resistance. *Clin Microbiol Rev* 1998;11:382-402.

Chapter **11**

Candidiasis

Candida species are ubiquitous fungi and the most common fungal pathogens affecting humans. The growing problem of mucosal and systemic candidiasis reflects the enormous increase in the pool of patients at risk and the increased opportunity for *Candida* species to invade tissues normally resistant to invasion. *Candida* species are true opportunistic pathogens that exploit recent technological advances to gain access to the vascular circulation and deep tissues. *Candida*, in particular, affects high-risk patients who are either immunocompromised or critically ill.

Epidemiology

The increased prevalence of local and systemic disease caused by *Candida* species has resulted in numerous clinical syndromes, the expression of which primarily depends on the host's immune status. *Candida* species produce a wide spectrum of diseases, ranging from superficial infections to invasive diseases such as hepatosplenic candidiasis (HSC), *Candida* peritonitis, and systemic candidiasis. Management of serious and life-threatening invasive candidiasis remains severely hampered by delays in diagnosis because of a lack of reliable diagnostic methods that would allow detection of fungemia and tissue invasion by *Candida* species.

Candida species are the most common cause of fungal infection affecting immunocompromised patients. Oropharyngeal colonization is found in 30% to 55% of healthy young adults, and *Candida* species may be detected in 40% to 65% of normal fecal flora.

Clinical and autopsy studies have confirmed the marked increase in the incidence of disseminated candidiasis, reflecting a parallel increase in the occurrence of candidemia. This increase is multifactorial in origin and reflects increased recognition as well as a growing population of patients at risk (ie, patients undergoing complex surgical procedures and those with indwelling vascular devices). The increase in disseminated candidiasis also reflects the improved survival of patients with underlying neoplasms, collagen vascular disease, and immunosuppression.

Candidiasis causes more fatalities than any other systemic mycosis.

In the febrile neutropenic patient who dies of sepsis, there is a 20% to 40% chance of finding evidence of invasive candidiasis at autopsy. Bodey described 21% of fatal infections in leukemic patients as the result of invasive fungal disease, in contrast with 13% and 6% of fatal infections in patients with lymphoma and solid tumors, respectively. Systemic candidiasis was described in 20% to 30% of patients undergoing bone marrow transplantation. In some university centers, *Candida* species are the second most common blood culture isolate. *Candida* species are now the fourth most commonly isolated pathogens from blood cultures in hospitals.

Candidemia and disseminated candidiasis mortality rates have not improved markedly over the past few years and remain in the 30% to 40% range. More than a decade ago, investigators reported the enormous economic impact of systemic candidiasis in hospitalized patients. Candidemia is associated with considerable prolongation of the length of hospital stay (70 days vs 40 days in patients who are comparable, matched, and nonfungemic). Although mucocutaneous fungal infections, such as oral thrush and *Candida e*sophagitis, are common in AIDS patients, candidemia and disseminated candidiasis are not.

Table 11-1: Significant *Candida* Species

Species Name		Isolation Rate
*C albicans**		50%-60%
C glabrata–less susceptible to all fluconazole, AMB*		15%-20%
C parapsilosis–catheter related*		10%-20%
*C tropicalis**		6%-12%
C krusei–"neutropenics"; intrinsic azole resistance, less susceptible to AMB*		1%-3%
C guilliermondii	AMB resistance	
C lusitaniae	AMB resistance	
C dubliniensis–primarily in HIV patients		

*Susceptible to voriconazole (Vfend®), posaconazole (Noxafil®)
AMB = amphotericin B

Microbiology

Candida species are yeast-like fungi that can form true hyphae and pseudohyphae. *Candida* species are typically confined to human and animal reservoirs; however, they are frequently recovered from the hospital environment, including food, countertops, air-conditioning vents, floors, respirators, and medical personnel. They are also normal commensals of diseased skin and mucosal surfaces of the gastrointestinal (GI), genitourinary, and respiratory tracts.

More than 100 species of *Candida* exist, but only a few are recognized as causing disease in humans. The medically significant *Candida* species are shown in Table 11-1. *Candida glabrata* and *Candida albicans* account for 70% to 80% of yeasts isolated from patients with invasive candidiasis.

Candida glabrata has recently become important because of its increasing worldwide incidence. It is intrinsically less susceptible to azoles and amphotericin B (Amphocin®, Fungizone®). Two uncommon *Candida* species, *Candida lusitaniae* and *Candida guilliermondii*, are important because of their innate resistance to amphotericin B. Another important *Candida* species is *Candida krusei*; although not as common as some *Candida* species, it is clinically significant because of its intrinsic resistance to fluconazole (Diflucan®), and it is less susceptible to all other antifungals, including amphotericin B. Posaconazole (Noxafil®), however, has displayed in-vitro activity against *C krusei*, *C glabrata*, and fluconazole-resistant *C albicans*. The susceptibility patterns of these *Candida* species are listed in Table 11-2.

Some uncommon non-*albicans Candida* species are associated with diseases in humans (Table 11-3).

Host Defense Mechanisms

As with most fungal infections, host defects play a significant role in the development of candidal infections. The intact skin constitutes a highly effective, impermeable barrier to *Candida* penetration. Disruption of the skin from burns, wounds, and ulceration permits invasion by colonizing opportunistic organisms. Similarly, indwelling intravascular devices provide an efficient conduit that bypasses the skin barrier. The major defense mechanisms operating at the mucosal level to maintain colonization and prevent invasion include the normal protective bacterial flora and cell-mediated immunity. The importance of the latter mechanism is highlighted by chronic mucocutaneous candidiasis with a congenital *Candida* antigen-specific deficiency, manifested by chronic, intractable, and severe mucocutaneous infection. However, candidemia and disseminated candidiasis are very rare in the presence of an intact humoral and phagocytic system. How the intact cell-mediated immune system prevents mucositis and mucosal invasion is still unclear.

Table 11-2: General Patterns of Susceptibility of *Candida* Species

***Candida* Species**	**Fluconazole (Diflucan®)**	**Itraconazole (Sporanox®)**
C albicans	S	S
C tropicalis	S	S
C parapsilosis	S	S
C glabrata	S-DD to R	S-DD to R
C krusei	R	S-DD to R
C lusitaniae	S	S
C kefyr	S	S
C guilliermondii	S	S
C dubliniensis	S	S

S = susceptible; R = resistant;
S-DD = susceptible-dose dependent

An effective phagocytic system is the critical defense mechanism that prevents *Candida* deep-tissue invasion, thereby limiting candidemia and preventing dissemination. Leukocyte failure includes quantitative reduction, usually as a result of acute leukemia or bone marrow failure, or following chemotherapy and marrow transplantation. Numerous host defects are generally associated with candidal infections. Polymorphonuclear and monocytic cells are capable of ingesting and killing blastospores and hyphal phases of *Candida*, a process that is enhanced by serum complement and specific immunoglobulins. Severe leukocyte qualitative dysfunction (eg, chronic

Flucytosine (Ancobon®)	Amphotericin B (Amphocin®, Fungizone®)	Echinocandins
S	S	S
S	S	S
S	S	S-I
S	S-I	S
I-R	S-I	S
S	S to R	S
S	S	S
S	S-R	I
S	S	S

11

granulomatous disease) is associated with disseminated, often life-threatening candidal infection. Myeloperoxidase deficiency also results in increased susceptibility to invasive infection.

Candida species also contain their own well-recognized virulence factors. Although not well characterized, several virulence factors may contribute to their ability to cause infection. The main virulence factors are surface molecules that permit adherence of the organism to other structures (human cells, extracellular matrix, prosthetic devices), acid proteases, phospholipase, and the ability to convert to a hyphal form.

Table 11-3: Characteristics and Disease States Associated With Uncommon Non-*albicans Candida* Species

Candida species	Characteristics/Disease States
C famata (*Torulopsis candida*)	Candidemia, endophthalmitis, peritonitis due to CAPD
C inconspicua	Candidemia in neutropenic patients; oropharyngeal, esophageal, and vaginal candidiasis in diabetic or HIV-positive patients
C lipolytica	Low virulence, catheter-related candidemia, commonly colonizes the stool, sputum, and mouth, although not associated with mucosal infections
C norvegensis	Recovered from the gastrointestinal and respiratory tracts, rarely causes candidemia and peritonitis
C pelliculosa Teleomorph: *Pichia anomala*	The most frequent of the uncommon causes of candidiasis; >20 cases of invasive candidiasis, including candidemia, endocarditis, intra-abdominal abscess, pyelonephritis, cerebral ventriculitis
C rugosa (*Monilia rugosa*)	Associated with nosocomial candidemia and invasive candidiasis in patients with burns, neutropenia, or catheter-associated infections

CAPD = continuous ambulatory peritoneal dialysis; MIC = minimum inhibitory concentration; R = resistant; S = susceptible; S-DD = susceptible-dose dependent

In vitro susceptibilities

AMB	5-FC	Flz	Itz	Clz	Ktz
S	S	S	S	S	S
S		R	R		
S	S	S	S	S	S
S	S	S-DD to R	S		S
Broad range of MICs S to R		S	S	S	S
S	S	Broad range of MICs S to S-DD	S		S

AMB = amphotericin B; Clz = clotrimazole (Lotrimin®); 5-FC = flucytosine; Flz = fluconazole; Itz = itraconazole; Ktz = ketoconazole (Nizoral®)

continued on next page

Table 11-3: Characteristics and Disease States Associated With Uncommon Non-*albicans Candida* Species *(continued)*

***Candida* species**	**Characteristics/Disease States**
C utilis (*Pichia jadinii*)	Used primarily in industry; a rare cause with only two cases of invasive candidiasis
C viswanathii	Recovered from respiratory tract and rare cause of meningitis
C zeylanoides	Low virulence, associated with catheter-related infections and septic arthritis

Pathogenesis

The first step in the development of *Candida* infections is colonization of the oropharynx and GI tract. Candidal colonization is at the highest levels in patients at the extremes of age, neonates, and adults older than 65 years. Numerous factors are associated with increased colonization. Once the colonized oropharyngeal mucosal surface is disrupted by chemotherapy or trauma, organisms penetrate the injured areas and gain access to the blood stream. Although the blastospore phase of *Candida* is capable of penetrating intact mucosal cells, the more virulent hyphal phase is more often associated with tissue invasion. Indwelling catheters appear to be a common route of blood stream invasion. This route is thought to account for at least 20% of candidemias. In prospective studies, fungemia has been found in 10% to 20% of all patients receiving intravenous (IV) hyperalimentation (total parenteral nutrition, or TPN) by way of central replaceable lines. Hyperalimentation

In vitro susceptibilities					
AMB	**5-FC**	**Flz**	**Itz**	**Clz**	**Ktz**
S		S			
S		S	S		

constitutes an independent risk factor, adding to the risk of the central IV line. The risk of fungemia is increased with prolonged duration of catheterization, which also increases the risk of local phlebitis, occasionally progressing to suppurative thrombosis. This seems to be a particular problem in patients with severe burns when other vascular access sites may be unavailable. In contrast, tunneled catheters (eg, Hickman and Broviac catheters) are rarely the source of candidemia, but the intravascular portion may become colonized and infected as the result of candidemia originating from a second independent focus or portal of entry. Fungal invasion from colonized wounds occurs rarely, except in patients with extensive burns. Similarly, the respiratory tract, although frequently colonized, is not a common site for *Candida* invasion and rarely is a source of dissemination.

Tissue invasion and candidemia are further facilitated by factors that alter the host's immune status. Several authors have noted the association between numbers of sites colonized with *Candida*, quantitative cultures obtained from these sites, and the occurrence of invasive *Candida* infections in granulocytopenic patients. Following invasion of the blood stream, efficient phagocytic cell function rapidly clears the invading organisms, especially when the inoculum is small. More prolonged candidemia is likely in granulocytopenic patients, especially when diagnosis and treatment are delayed, resulting in increased risk of hematogenous spread and metastatic seeding of multiple visceral sites, primarily the kidneys, eyes, liver, skin and central nervous system. Manifestations of metastatic infection may be apparent immediately or may be delayed several weeks or even months, long after predisposing factors (eg, granulocytopenia) have resolved.

A third route for blood stream invasion is persorption via the GI wall, following massive colonization with a high titer of organisms that pass directly into the blood stream. Candidemia and disseminated candidiasis almost invariably follow serious bacterial infections, especially bacteremia. Although simultaneous bacteremia and fungemia are occasionally reported and associated with a high mortality, the sequential relationship between the two infections is unexplained. Antimicrobial agents have no direct effect on the invasive capacity of *Candida* but do enhance mucosal and skin colonization.

In contrast to patients with candidemia and systemic candidiasis, a more localized form of visceral candidiasis is observed involving only the liver or spleen. This syndrome has been called focal hepatic candidiasis or HSC and is most often seen in association with acute myeloblastic leukemia, particularly after cytosine arabinoside therapy. Hepatic involvement is thought to follow GI ulceration induced by chemotherapy in individuals with bowel colonization with *Candida*, and the yeast may reach the liver via the portal venous system.

Candida infections can present in a wide spectrum of clinical syndromes, depending on the type of infection and the degree of immunosuppression.

Cutaneous Candidiasis Syndromes

Generalized Cutaneous Candidiasis

This is an unusual form of cutaneous candidiasis that manifests as a diffuse eruption over the trunk, thorax, and extremities. Patients have a history of generalized pruritus that increases in severity in the genitocrural folds, anal region, axillae, hands, and feet. Physical examination reveals a widespread rash that begins as individual vesicles and spreads into large confluent areas.

Intertrigo

Patients generally have a history of intertrigo affecting any site where skin surfaces are in close proximity, providing a warm and moist environment. Generally, a red pruritic rash develops that begins with vesiculopustules and then enlarges, followed by rupture of the bullae, causing maceration and fissuring. The area involved has a scalloped border, with a white rim consisting of necrotic epidermis that surrounds the erythematous macerated base. Satellite lesions are frequently found and may coalesce and extend into larger lesions.

Candida Folliculitis

This infection is predominantly found in hair follicles and rarely becomes extensive.

Erosio Interdigitalis Blastomycetica

The patient often has a history of *Candida* infection, with a painful rash between the toes and fingers. Physical examination reveals a tender, erythematous eruption with a red base that frequently extends onto the sides of the digits.

Paronychia and Onychomycosis

These infections are frequently associated with immersion of the hands in water and patients with diabetes mellitus. Patients have a history of a painful and erythematous area around and underneath the nail and the nailbed. Physical examination reveals inflammation that becomes warm, glistening, tense, and erythematous and may extend extensively under the nail, with secondary nail thickening, ridging, discoloration, and occasional nail loss.

Chronic Mucocutaneous Candidiasis

CMC describes *Candida* infections of the skin, hair, nails, and mucous membranes that tend to have a protracted and persistent course. Most infections begin in infancy or the first 2 decades of life; onset in people older than 30 years is rare. These chronic and recurrent infections frequently result in a disfiguring form called *Candida* granuloma. Most patients survive for long periods and rarely experience disseminated fungal infections. The most common cause of death is bacterial and not *Candida* sepsis. CMC is frequently associated with multiple endocrinopathies. Physical examination reveals disfiguring lesions of the face, scalp, hands, and nails (Figure 11-1; see color plate insert), occasionally associated with oral thrush and vitiligo.

Mucosal Candidiasis

Oropharyngeal Candidiasis

Candida colonization of the oropharynx is present in 20% to 55% of normal adults and increases dramatically in debilitated and immunocompromised hosts. It is most prevalent in infants, the elderly, and immunocompromised patients. Oropharyngeal candidiasis (OPC) occurs in association with serious underlying conditions such as diabetes, leukemia, neoplasia, steroid use, antimicrobial therapy, radiation therapy, dentures, and HIV infection. Persistent OPC in infants may be the first manifestation of childhood AIDS or chronic mucocutaneous candidiasis. Somonis and Bodey reported that 28% of cancer patients not receiving antifungal prophylaxis developed OPC. In a similar immunocompromised hospitalized population, Yeo observed OPC in 57% of patients.

Approximately 80% to 90% of patients with HIV infection will develop OPC at some stage of their disease.

The presence of OPC should alert the physician to the possibility of underlying HIV infection. Sixty percent of untreated HIV-positive patients develop an AIDS-related infection or Kaposi's sarcoma within 2 years of the appearance of OPC. Profound differences exist between HIV-positive and HIV-negative patient populations that influence the natural history, diagnosis, and management of mucosal candidiasis. In addition, prospective studies indicate that the microbiology of mucosal candidiasis is changing. Recently, there has been a significant increase in the incidence of non-*albicans Candida* species recovered from HIV-positive patients. Many HIV-positive patients experience recurrent episodes of OPC and esophageal candidiasis as HIV progresses, and they ultimately receive numerous courses of antifungals that may contribute to the development of antifungal resistance. Antifungal agents are less effective and take longer to achieve a clinical response in HIV-positive patients than in cancer patients.

Candida albicans remains the most common species responsible for OPC cases (80% to 90%). The ability of *C albicans* to adhere to buccal epithelial cells is critical in establishing oral colonization. *Candida albicans* adheres better in vitro to epithelial cells than non-*albicans Candida* species. Following colonization, *Candida* may persist for months or years in low numbers without manifestations. The low numbers of colonizing organisms are the result of effective antifungal host defense mechanisms in the oral cavity. Low salivary flow rates correlate with higher prevalence rate of *Candida*.

The manifestations of thrush vary significantly, from none to a sore, painful mouth, burning tongue, and dysphagia. Frequently, severe objective changes are asymptomatic. Clinical signs include a diffuse erythema with white patches that appear as discrete lesions on the surfaces of the mucosa, throat, tongue, and gums (Figure 11-2; see color plate insert). With some difficulty, the plaques can be wiped off, revealing a raw, erythematous, and sometimes bleeding base.

OPC can impair quality of life and result in a reduction in fluid or food intake. The most serious complication of untreated OPC is extension to the esophagus. Fungemia and disseminated candidiasis are uncommon.

Oropharyngeal candidiasis has five clinical forms.

(1) Acute pseudomembranous candidiasis (exudative) is the most common form, especially in HIV-positive patients, and presents with whitish-yellow, thick, curd-like discharge on mucosal surfaces. Lesions may be small and discrete or confluent, involving the entire oral mucosa.

(2) Chronic atrophic stomatitis–denture stomatitis is a very common form of OPC that is frequently asymptomatic, but patients may complain of soreness and burning of the mouth. The characteristic signs are chronic erythema and edema of the portion of the palate that comes into contact with dentures. Denture stomatitis was found in 24% to 60% of denture wearers and is more common in women than in men. The association between *Candida* and denture stomatitis is now well documented, with the detection of *Candida* by culture or microscopy in more than 90% of subjects. Even without signs or symptoms, the prevalence of oral yeast is invariably higher in denture wearers. Maximum concentrations of yeast are found on the denture-fitting surface. *Candida* species readily adhere to plastic objects such as orthodontic appliances. Given the lack of fungal invasion and the lack of exudative features characteristic of oral thrush, the pathogenesis remains unclear. Notably, *C glabrata* has been identified in 15%

to 30% of all cultures, a higher prevalence than generally found in the mouth.

(3) Angular cheilitis (perlèche), also called cheilosis, is characterized by soreness, erythema, and fissuring at the corners of the mouth. Cheilitis may accompany oral thrush or denture stomatitis, or may appear in the absence of oral disease. Vitamin deficiency and iron-deficiency anemia are also associated with cheilitis, but they alone do not provide a direct cause-effect relationship. Angular cheilitis frequently responds to topical antifungals.

(4) Chronic hyperplastic candidiasis (*Candida* leukoplakia) produces oral white patches, or leukoplakia, that are discrete, transparent-to-whitish, raised lesions of variable sizes found on the inner surface of the cheeks and, less frequently, on the tongue. These lesions are found predominantly in men and are strongly associated with smoking. Most examples of leukoplakia are not related to *Candida* infection; however, *Candida* invasion of the lesions has been observed in 60% to 90% of biopsies. Although leukoplakia lesions are thought to be premalignant, there is no known association between *Candida* and either dysplasia or cancer. Although leukoplakia sometimes responds to prolonged topical therapy with antimycotics, most lesions do not and instead require diagnostic biopsy and surgical resection.

(5) Midline glossitis (median rhomboid glossitis, acute atrophic stomatitis) refers to symmetrical lesions of the center dorsum of the tongue characterized by loss of papillae and erythema. Based on isolation of *Candida* from these lesions, it has been suspected that *Candida* is responsible for the syndrome rather than an innocent bystander. The pathologic role of *Candida* in this syndrome remains unresolved despite occasional histologic smears showing *Candida* hyphae invading tissues.

Esophageal Candidiasis

In contrast to the skin and oral mucosa, where infection is common, the esophagus is an uncommon site of infection. *Candida* esophagitis invariably occurs in predisposed individuals. *Candida albicans* is the most common cause of esophagitis and, after the oropharynx, the esophagus is the most common site of GI candidiasis. The prevalence of *Candida* esophagitis has increased because of AIDS and the increased pool of transplant patients, cancer patients, and severely immunocompromised patients.

Candida microorganisms are frequently recovered from the esophageal surface and reach the esophagus in oral secretions. In contrast to oral candidiasis, little is known about host and yeast factors operative in the pathogenesis of esophageal candidiasis. Experimental models have not been established, but it is likely that the usual yeast virulence factors and defects in host defense mechanism operate.

Esophageal candidiasis in an HIV-positive patient may be the first manifestation of AIDS. In cancer patients, factors predisposing to esophagitis include previous exposure to radiation, recent cytotoxic chemotherapy, antibiotic therapy, corticosteroid therapy, and neutropenia. The high prevalence of esophagitis in AIDS patients indicates the critical role of cell-mediated immunity in normally protecting the esophagus from *Candida* invasion. *Candida* esophagitis tends to occur later in the natural history of HIV infection and almost invariably at a much lower CD4 count.

Candida esophagitis presents most commonly with dysphagia, odynophagia, and retrosternal pain. Constitutional findings, including fever, occur only occasionally. Rarely, epigastric pain is the dominant symptom. Even before AIDS, a male-to-female predominance was noted. Most patients have underlying hematologic cancers or HIV infection or have undergone recent transplantation. Although esophagitis may occur as an extension of OPC, in more than two thirds of published reports, the esophagus was the only site involved, and it was reported more often in the distal two thirds than in the proximal one third of the esophagus. An occasional feature of *Candida* esophagitis in AIDS patients is the absence of symptoms despite extensive objective esophageal involvement. Physical findings vary in distribution, character, and severity. Kodsi classified *Candida e*sophagitis on the basis of its endoscopic appearance. Type I cases refer to a few white or beige plaques up to 2 mm in diameter. Type II plaques are larger and more numerous. In the milder grades, plaques may be hyperemic or edematous, but there is no ulceration. Type III plaques may be confluent, linear, nodular, and elevated, with hyperemia and frank ulceration, and type IV plaques additionally have increased friability of the mucosa and occasional narrowing of the lumen.

Uncommon complications of esophagitis include perforation, aortic-esophageal fistula formation, and, rarely, extensive necrosis that destroys the esophageal mucosa. In neutropenic patients, *Candida* esophagitis may lead to candidemia and disseminated candidiasis and, when extensive ulceration is present, may provide a portal of
entry for bacteria that cause bacteremia.

A reliable diagnosis can only be made by histologic evidence of tissue invasion in biopsy material. Nevertheless, antifungal therapy is frequently initiated empirically with minimal criteria in a high-risk patient. The mere presence of *Candida* within an esophageal lesion as established by brushings, smear, or culture does not provide sufficient evidence to distinguish *Candida* as a commensal from *Candida* as an invasive pathogen. While esophageal brushings are highly sensitive in diagnosing esophagitis, specificity is not high and neither is the positive predictive value. The presence of *Candida* hyphae in esophageal brushings is just as compatible with colonization as it is with infection.

In the absence of biopsy material, radiologic features previously formed the basis for diagnosis. A barium contrast upper GI x-ray in *Candida* esophagitis may reveal shaggy mucosal irregularities and nodular filling defects. As severity increases, the nodular pattern becomes extensive, giving a cobblestone appearance. Peristaltic abnormalities are also common. Infrequently, discrete ulceration and stenosis may occur. Unfortunately, the sensitivity of barium swallow is relatively low, and radiologic abnormalities are often absent in mild to moderate esophagitis, especially in patients with AIDS. Accordingly, radiology has been replaced by endoscopy, which not only provides a rapid and highly sensitive diagnosis, but also is the only reliable method of differentiating among the various causes of esophagitis. The characteristic endoscopic appearance is described as yellow-white plaques on an erythematous background, with varying degrees of ulceration. White plaques and pseudomembranes are not exclusive to *Candida* infection, but erythema in the absence of plaques may be due to *Candida*.

Differential diagnosis includes radiation esophagitis, reflux esophagitis, cytomegalovirus, or herpes simplex virus infection. In the AIDS patient, it is not uncommon to identify more than one etiologic agent causing esophagitis.

Respiratory Tract Candidiasis

Laryngeal candidiasis: This is an uncommon form, but it may be a source for disseminated candidiasis. Laryngeal candidiasis is seen primarily in HIV-positive patients and occasionally in hematologic cancers. The patient may present with a sore throat and hoarseness. Physical examination generally is unremarkable, and the diagnosis is made by direct or indirect laryngoscopy.

***Candida* tracheobronchitis:** This is a rare form of candidiasis. Most patients with *Candida* tracheobronchitis are HIV positive or severely immunocompromised, complaining of fever, productive cough, and shortness of breath. Physical examination reveals dyspnea and scattered rhonchi. The diagnosis generally is made during bronchoscopy.

***Candida* pneumonia:** This is also a rare form of candidiasis. The most common form of infection appears to be multiple lung abscesses due to the hematogenous dissemination of *Candida* species. The high degree of colonization and isolation of *Candida* species from the respiratory tract makes it difficult to make a diagnosis. The diagnosis requires the visualization of *Candida* invasion on histopathology. The patient's history reveals similar risk factors for disseminated candidiasis, and patients complain of shortness of breath, cough, and respiratory distress. Physical examination reveals fever, dyspnea, and variable breath sounds from clear to rhonchi to scattered rales.

Vulvovaginal Candidiasis

In the United States, *Candida* vaginitis is the second most common vaginal infection. During the childbearing years, 75% of women experience at least one episode of vulvovaginal candidiasis (VVC), and 40% to 50% of these women experience a second episode. A small subpopulation of women experiences repeated, recurrent episodes of *Candida* vaginitis. *Candida* may be isolated from the genital tract of about 10% to 20% of asymptomatic, healthy women of childbearing age.

Candida vaginitis can be classified as complicated or uncomplicated, depending on factors such as severity and frequency of infection and the causative *Candida* species (Table 11-4).

Asymptomatic colonization with *Candida* is common. *Candida* organisms gain access to the vaginal lumen and then adhere to vaginal epithelial cells. Several factors are associated with increased rates of asymptomatic vaginal colonization with *Candida* as well as *Candida* vaginitis, including pregnancy (30% to 40%), use of oral contraceptives with a high estrogen content, and uncontrolled diabetes mellitus. The hormonal dependence of the infection is illustrated by the fact that *Candida* is seldom isolated from premenarchal girls, and the prevalence of *Candida* vaginitis is lower after menopause, except in women taking hormone replacement therapy (HRT). Other factors include uncontrolled diabetes mellitus, corticosteroid and antimicrobial therapy, use of an intrauterine device, high frequency of coitus, and refined-sugar eating binges.

Pathogenesis: Germination of *Candida* enhances colonization and tissue invasion. Factors that enhance or facilitate germination (eg, HRT, pregnancy) tend to precipitate symptomatic vaginitis; measures that inhibit germination (eg, bacterial flora) may prevent acute vaginitis in women who are asymptomatic carriers of yeast. During pregnancy, the incidence of clinical attacks reaches a maximum in the third trimester, but symptomatic recurrences are more common throughout pregnancy. It is generally thought that high levels of reproductive hormones raise the glycogen content in the vagina and provide a carbon source for *Candida* growth and germination. Estrogens enhance vaginal epithelial cell avidity for *Candida* adherence, and a yeast cytosol receptor or binding system for female reproductive hormones has been documented. In addition, estrogens enhance yeast-mycelial transformation. Low-estrogen oral contraceptives may also cause an increase in *Candida* vaginitis. HRT may contribute to vaginitis in postmenopausal women.

Vaginal colonization is more common in diabetes, while uncontrolled diabetes may predispose to symptomatic vaginitis.

Symptomatic VVC is often observed during or after use of antibiotics. Although no antimicrobial agent is free of this complication, the broad-spectrum antibiotics (eg, tetracyclines, ampicillin, cephalosporins) are mainly responsible; they are thought to act by eliminating the normal protective vaginal bacterial flora. *Lactobacillus* species in the natural flora provide a colonization-resistance mechanism and prevent germination of *Candida*. However, most women taking antibiotics do not develop *Candida* vaginitis.

Environmental factors that predispose to *Candida* vaginitis include tight, poorly ventilated clothing and ny-

Table 11-4: Classification of *Candida* Vaginitis

Feature	Uncomplicated	Complicated
Severity	Mild or moderate	Severe
Frequency	Sporadic	Recurrent
Organism	*Candida albicans*	Non-*albicans* species of *Candida*
Host	Normal	Abnormal (eg, uncontrolled diabetes mellitus)

lon underclothing, which increase perineal moisture and temperature. Chemical contact, local allergy, and hypersensitivity reactions also predispose to symptomatic vaginitis. In patients who are debilitated or immunosuppressed, oral and vaginal candidiasis correlate with reduced cell-mediated immunity. This is evident in chronic mucocutaneous candidiasis and AIDS.

Recurrent and chronic *Candida* vaginitis: Various theories have been proposed to explain recurrent vaginitis. The intestinal reservoir theory is based on the recovery of *Candida* on rectal culture in almost 100% of women with VVC. However, other studies have shown a lower concordance between rectal and vaginal cultures in patients with recurrent VVC. The sexual transmission theory is based on penile colonization with *Candida*, which is present in about 20% of male partners of women with recurrent VVC. Infected partners usually carry identical strains. Oral colonization of partners with an identical strain of *Candida* also occurs and may be a source of orogenital transmission. However, in most studies involving treatment of partners, there was no reduction in the frequency of episodes of vaginitis. According to the vaginal relapse theory, although antimycotic therapy may reduce the number of *Candida* in the lumen and alleviate signs and symptoms of inflammation, the eradication of *Candida* from the vaginal mucosa is incomplete because the antimycotic agents are fungistatic. The small numbers of organisms that persist in the vagina result in continued carriage of the organism; thus, when host environmental conditions permit, the colonizing organisms increase and undergo mycelial transformation, resulting in a new clinical episode. Drug resistance is seldom responsible for recurrent VVC in women infected with *C albicans*. A final theory is based on reduced host resistance, which includes qualitative and quantitative deficiency in the normal protective vaginal bacterial flora and an acquired, often transient, antigen-specific deficiency in T lymphocyte function that permits unchecked yeast proliferation and germination.

Clinical features: Vulvar pruritus is the most common symptom of VVC and is present in most symptomatic patients. Vaginal discharge is often minimal and occasionally absent. Although described as being typically 'cottage cheese-like' in character, the discharge may vary from watery to homogeneously thick. Vaginal soreness, irritation, vulvar burning, dyspareunia, and external dysuria are common. If there is an odor, it is minimal. Characteristically, symptoms are exacerbated during the week before the onset of menses, while the onset of menstrual flow frequently brings some relief.

Examination reveals erythema and swelling of the labia and vulva, often with discrete pustulopapular peripheral lesions (Figures 11-3 and 11-4; see color plate insert). The cervix is normal. Vaginal mucosal erythema with adherent whitish discharge is present.

Diagnosis: In most symptomatic patients, VVC is readily diagnosed by microscopic examination of vaginal secretions. A wet mount of saline preparation has a sensitivity of only 40% to 60%. A 10% potassium hydroxide preparation is more sensitive in diagnosing the presence of germinated yeast. Patients with *Candida* vaginitis have a normal vaginal pH (4.0 to 4.5). A pH of more than 4.5 suggests bacterial vaginosis, trichomoniasis, or mixed infection. Routine cultures are unnecessary, but in suspicious cases, vaginal culture should be performed with negative microscopy. Although vaginal culture is the most sensitive method available for detecting *Candida*, a positive culture does not necessarily indicate that *Candida* is responsible for the vaginal symptoms. Commercial tests (including latex agglutination slide tests) are less sensitive than culture and have no advantages over microscopy. Newer assays using *Candida*-specific DNA probes and polymerase chain reactions are available, but they are still investigational and expensive.

Urinary Tract Candidiasis

Candiduria is rare in otherwise healthy people. Although epidemiologic studies have documented candiduria in approximately 10% of individuals sampled, many of these culture results reverted to negative when a clean-catch technique was used. The incidence of fungal urinary tract infections (UTIs), specifically candiduria, has dramatically increased recently, especially among patients with indwelling Foley catheters.

A study by Platt et al demonstrated that 26.5% of all urinary tract infections related to indwelling catheters were caused by fungi. *Candida* species are the organisms most frequently isolated from the urine samples of patients in surgical intensive care units (ICUs); 10% to 15% of nosocomial UTIs are caused by *Candida* species.

Risk factors: Diabetes mellitus may predispose patients to candiduria by enhancing *Candida* colonization of the vulvovestibular area (in women), by enhancing urinary fungal growth in the presence of glycosuria, by lowering host resistance to invasion by fungi as a consequence of impaired phagocytic activity, and by promoting stasis of urine in a neurogenic bladder.

Antibiotics also increase colonization of the GI tract by *Candida* species, which are normally present in ~30% of immunocompetent adults. However, among patients who are receiving antibiotics, colonization rates approach 100%. Because there is little evidence that systemic antibiotics directly influence *Candida* species proliferation or virulence, it is likely that antibiotics contribute to colonization by *Candida* species by suppressing endogenous bacterial flora, primarily in the gut and lower genital tract and possibly in superficial areas adjacent to the urethral meatus. Candiduria is almost invariably preceded by bacteriuria.

Indwelling urinary catheters serve as a portal of entry for microorganisms into the urinary drainage system. All catheters become colonized if left in place long enough.

Other risk factors include the extremes of age, female sex, use of immunosuppressive agents, venous catheters, interruption of urine flow, radiation therapy, and genitourinary tuberculosis.

Most fungal infections of the urinary tract involve *Candida* species. In a large multicenter study by Kauffman and colleagues, *C albicans* was found in 51.8% of 861 patients with funguria. The second most common pathogen (134 patients) was *C glabrata*. Risk factors for *C glabrata* UTI are similar to those that predispose a patient to *C albicans* infection. Virtually all epidemiologic studies have concluded that, although *C albicans* is the most common species encountered, non-*albicans Candida* species are also very common and far more prevalent than in other sites (ie, oropharynx and vagina), possibly as a function of urine composition and pH selectivity for non-*albicans* species. In approximately 10% of patients, more than one species of *Candida* are found simultaneously.

Ascending infection is by far the most common route for infection of the bladder. It occurs more often in women because of a shorter urethra and frequent vulvovestibular colonization with *Candida* (10% to 35%). Ascending infection that originates in the bladder can infrequently lead to infection of the upper urinary tract, especially if vesicoureteral reflux or obstruction of urinary flow occurs. This may eventually result in acute pyelonephritis and, rarely, candidemia. A fungus ball consisting of yeast, hyphal elements, epithelial and inflammatory cells, and, sometimes, renal medullary tissue secondary to papillary necrosis may complicate ascending or descending infections. The fungus ball tends to be found in dilated areas of the urinary tract, especially in the bladder in the presence of obstruction.

Hematogenous spread is the most common route for renal infection (ie, renal candidiasis). *Candida* species may have a tropism for the kidneys; one study revealed that 90% of patients with fatal disseminated candidiasis had renal involvement at autopsy. Isolated hematogenous renal infection can occur after transient candidemia. Frequently, when renal candidiasis is suspected, blood cultures are no longer positive.

Diagnosis: The finding of *Candida* organisms in the urine may represent contamination, colonization of the drainage device, or infection. Contamination of a urine specimen is common, especially with suboptimal urine collection from a catheterized patient or from a woman who has heavy yeast colonization of the vulvovestibular area. Given the capacity of yeast to grow in urine, small numbers of yeast cells that migrate into the collected urine sample may quickly multiply. Therefore, high colony counts could be the result of yeast contamination or colonization. Colonization usually refers to the asymptomatic adherence and settlement of yeast, usually on drainage catheters or other foreign bodies in the urinary tract (ie, stents and nephrostomy tubes), and it may result in a high concentration of the organisms on urine culture. Simply culturing the organism does not imply clinical significance, regardless of the concentration of organisms in the urine. Accordingly, some clinicians require confirmation of

Candida presence by a second urine sample examination before they initiate treatment or further investigation. Infection is caused by superficial or deep tissue invasion. Kozinn showed that colony counts of $>10^4$ colony-forming units (cfu)/mL of urine were associated with infection in patients without indwelling urinary catheters, although clinically significant renal candidiasis has been reported with colony counts of 10^3 cfu/mL of urine. Pyuria supports the diagnosis of infection in patients with a urinary catheter. Pyuria can result from mechanical injury of the bladder mucosa by the catheter or from coexistent bacteriuria. In summary, absence of pyuria and low colony counts tend to rule out *Candida* infection, but the low specificity of pyuria and counts $>10^3$ cfu/mL require that results be interpreted in the clinical context. The number of yeast cells in urine has little value in localizing the anatomical level of infection. Rarely, a granular cast containing *Candida* hyphal elements is found in urine that localizes the infection to renal parenchyma. Declining renal function suggests urinary obstruction or renal invasion. For candiduria patients with sepsis, is it not only necessary to obtain blood cultures, but also, given the frequency with which obstruction and stasis coexist, essential to perform radiographic visualization of the upper tract. Any febrile patient for whom therapy for candiduria is considered necessary should be investigated for the anatomic source of candiduria. In contrast, patients without sepsis require no additional studies unless candiduria persists after the removal of catheters.

Clinical manifestations: Candiduria is most often asymptomatic and occurs in hospitalized or nursing home patients with indwelling catheters. These patients usually show none of the signs or symptoms associated with UTI. Symptomatic *Candida* cystitis is uncommon and characterized by bladder irritation, dysuria, hematuria, frequency, urgency, and suprapubic tenderness. Cystoscopy, although rarely indicated unless a fungus ball is suspected or if ascending infection occurs, reveals soft, pearly white, elevated patches with friable mucosa underneath and hyperemia of the bladder mucosa. Symptomatic *Candida* cystitis is rare in catheterized patients, which implies that the bladder is relatively resistant to invasion by *Candida* species. Similarly, symptomatic *Candida* cystitis is rare in noncatheterized patients. Emphysematous cystitis is also a rare complication of lower UTI, whereas prostatic abscess caused by *Candida* species is common, especially among patients with diabetes.

Upper UTIs present with fever, leukocytosis, and costovertebral angle tenderness. On clinical grounds, ascending pyelonephritis and urosepsis with *Candida* species are, therefore, indistinguishable from bacterial pyelonephritis and urosepsis. Ascending infection almost invariably occurs in the presence of urinary obstruction and stasis, especially in patients with diabetes or nephrolithiasis. *Candida* pyelonephritis is often complicated by local suppurative disease, resulting in pyonephrosis as well as focal abscess formation, diagnosed by ultrasonography and computed tomography (CT) scan.

A major complication of upper UTI is obstruction caused by fungus balls (bezoars), which can also be visualized on ultrasonography. Renal colic may occur with the passage of fungal 'stones,' which are actually portions of fungus balls.

Patients with hematogenous seeding of the kidneys caused by candidemia may present with high fever, hemodynamic instability, and variable renal insufficiency. Blood culture results are positive for *Candida* in half of these patients. Retinal or skin involvement may suggest dissemination, but candiduria and a decline in renal function are often the only clues to systemic candidiasis in a febrile, high-risk patient.

Abdominal Candidiasis, Including Peritonitis

Candida infection has been increasingly recognized as a cause of abdominal sepsis and is associated with a high mortality. Peritoneal contamination with *Candida* species follows either spontaneous GI perforation or surgical opening of the gut. However, after contaminating the peritoneal cavity, *Candida* organisms do not inevitably result in peritonitis and clinical infection. Peritonitis is more likely to follow proliferation of accompanying bacterial pathogens, but it can occur with *Candida* alone. Several other risk factors have been recognized for peritonitis, including recent or concomitant antimicrobial therapy, inoculum size, and surgery for acute pancreatitis. Translocation of *Candida* across the intact intestinal mucosa has been shown experimentally in animals and in a volunteer. Additional risk factors for invasive candidiasis include diabetes, malnutrition, ischemia, hyperalimentation, neoplasia, and multiple abdominal surgeries. Pancreatic transplantation, especially with enteric drainage, is associated with intra-abdominal *Candida* abscess formation. *Candida* species have a unique affinity for the inflamed pancreas, resulting in intrapancreatic abscesses or infecting an accompanying pseudocyst. In *Candida* peritonitis, *Candida* usually remains localized to the peritoneal cavity, with the incidence of dissemination at about 25%.

The clinical significance of *Candida* isolated from the peritoneal cavity during or after surgery has been controversial. Several earlier studies concluded that a positive culture did not require antifungal therapy. Calandra et al, in a review of *Candida* isolates from the peritoneal cavity, determined that *Candida* caused intra-abdominal infection in 19 of 49 (39%) patients. In 61% of patients, *Candida* isolation occurred without signs of peritonitis. Accordingly, in each patient, clinicians should consider the clinical signs of infection and other risk factors when deciding whether to initiate antifungal therapy.

Candida peritonitis as a complication of continuous ambulatory peritoneal dialysis (CAPD) is more common, but it infrequently results in positive blood cultures and hematogenous dissemination. In a series of CAPD patients followed for 5 years, fungal peritonitis, most commonly

Candida species, accounted for 7% of episodes of peritonitis. Seventeen cases of fungal peritonitis were reported, with eight associated deaths. Few risk factors have emerged except for recent hospitalization, previous episodes of peritonitis, and antibacterial therapy. Clinically, fungal peritonitis cannot be differentiated from bacterial peritonitis except by gram stain and culture of dialysate.

Biliary Candidiasis

Yeast in the bile is not uncommon, especially after biliary surgery, and has the same significance as asymptomatic bactibilia (ie, colonization only). While yeast is a potential source of future infection, it is not justification for antifungal therapy. *Candida* is an infrequent cause of cholecystitis and cholangitis. Other risk factors include diabetes, immunosuppression, and abdominal malignancy. A major contributory factor is the use of biliary stents placed to overcome obstruction. In this setting, infection is usually polymicrobial and *Candida* is a pathogen that should not be ignored.

Cholecystitis due to *Candida* has been reported in patients with AIDS and cholangiopathy. Biliary candidiasis can be classified as uncomplicated or complicated. In uncomplicated cholecystitis, *Candida* organisms are confined to bile and the gallbladder without extrabiliary spread. In complicated cholecystitis, infection spreads to adjacent structures, including the liver and peritoneum. Uncomplicated disease has minimal mortality, and cure is frequently achieved by cholecystectomy.

Candida Osteomyelitis and Arthritis

Although previously rare, *Candida* osteomyelitis is now not uncommon. Most cases are the result of hematogenous dissemination, with seeding of long bones in children and the axial skeleton in adults. Sites of bone infection include the spine (vertebral and intravertebral disk), wrist, femur, humerus, and costochondral junctions.

Osteomyelitis may present weeks or months after the causal candidemic episode; therefore, at presentation, blood cultures are usually negative and radiologic findings nonspecific. Diagnosis usually requires a bone biopsy.

Occasionally, postoperative wound infections may spread to contiguous bone such as the sternum and to vertebrae. Regardless of the source, manifestations resemble bacterial infection but run a more insidious course, with a significant delay in diagnosis.

Hematogenous vertebral osteomyelitis usually (in 95% of patients) affects the lower thoracic or lumbar spine. In one series, 83% of patients complained of back pain for more than one month, 32% presented with fever, and 19% had associated neurologic complications. Blood cultures are positive in only 50% to 60% of cases.

Candida arthritis generally represents a complication of hematogenous candidiasis and rarely follows local trauma, surgery, or intra-articular injections. Patients with underlying joint disease (eg, rheumatoid arthritis, prosthetic joints) are at increased risk. *Candida* arthritis can occur in any joint and has been reported in multiple joints in up to 25% of cases. Most infections, however, are monoarticular and commonly involve the knee. Infection resembles bacterial septic arthritis, but chronic infection often develops with secondary bone involvement because of the delay in diagnosis and suboptimal treatment.

Candidemia and Disseminated Candidiasis

Rex et al have divided candidemia or systemic candidiasis into four groups or syndromes: catheter-related candidiasis, acute disseminated candidiasis, chronic disseminated candidiasis, and deep-organ candidiasis. Although hematogenous involvement occurs at some stage in the evolution of all four, only the first two are strongly associated with documented candidemia. Thus, use of candidemia as a marker of invasive candidiasis results in the underestimation of the true incidence of invasive candidiasis.

A dramatic increase in the incidence of candidemia has occurred in the last 4 decades, originating in tertiary care centers and now observed in virtually all hospitals. A published population-based survey reported that the incidence of nosocomial candidemia in the United States is 8 cases per 100,000 population. If defined on the basis of candidemia, the incidence of invasive candidiasis has a bimodal age distribution, with peaks at the extremes of age—75 cases per 100,000 population in infants younger than 1 year and 26 cases per 100,000 population in adults older than 65 years. *Candida* is the fourth most common cause of blood stream infections (BSI) in the United States. Epidemiologic data indicate that at least 72% of all nosocomial functions and 8% to 15% of all nosocomial BSI are caused by *Candida* species.

Within the hospital setting, the departments with the highest rates of candidemia include ICUs, surgical units, trauma units, and neonatal ICUs. In fact, 25% to 50% of all nosocomial candidemia occurs in critical care units. Neutropenic patients, who were formerly the highest risk group, are no longer the most vulnerable subpopulation because of the widespread use of fluconazole prophylaxis during neutropenia. In some tertiary care centers, *C albicans* is no longer the most common blood stream isolate, having been replaced by *C glabrata*, which has replaced *Candida tropicalis* as the most prevalent non-*albicans* species, now causing 3% to 35% of all candidemias. Non-*albicans Candida* species have also become an increasing problem in ICUs, attributed to the more widespread use of fluconazole in this population.

Risk factors for *Candida* blood stream infections include antibiotics, chemotherapy, corticosteroids, intravascular catheters, receipt of TPN, recent surgery, hospitalization in ICU, cancer, neutropenia, and fungal colonization. The most important risk factor for invasive candidiasis is a prolonged stay in the ICU. In a prospective study conducted in six surgical ICUs, multivariate analysis revealed increased risk with prior abdominal surgery (relative risk [RR] 7.3), acute renal failure (RR 4.2), TPN (RR 3.6), and triple-lumen catheter (RR 5.4). Surprisingly, in contrast to multiple other studies, prior fungal colonization was not shown to be a risk factor, and receiving any systemic antifungal was associated with reduced risk.

Clinical aspects of candidemia can vary significantly, including fever alone, absence of any organ-specific manifestations, or a wide spectrum of manifestations, including fulminant sepsis (Table 11-5). Accordingly, acute candidemia is indistinguishable from bacterial sepsis and septic shock. Clinical manifestations of fungemia are frequently superimposed on those because of the underlying pathology. In general, there are no specific clinical features associated with individual *Candida* species.

Candidemia may present with manifestations of systemic and invasive metastatic candidiasis, although when these occur, blood cultures have frequently become negative. Thus, candidemia is a marker, although insensitive to deeply invasive candidiasis. Only 50% of patients with disseminated candidiasis will have positive blood cultures, and an antemortem diagnosis is even lower (15% to 40%). Dissemination to multiple organs may occur with candidemia, especially to the kidney, eye, brain, myocardium, liver, and spleen in leukemia patients, but it can also involve the lungs, skin, vertebral column, and endocardium.

The possibility of asymptomatic disseminated infection drives the treatment principles of candidemia. Transient candidemia can occur from any source but most often follows intravascular catheter infection, with prompt resolution after catheter removal. Prolonged candidemia, especially when blood cultures remain persistently positive on appropriate antifungal treatment, suggests a persistent focus or source (eg, intravascular catheter, abscess, suppurative thrombophlebitis, endocarditis, severe neutropenia) or antifungal resistance, which is rare, but possible with

Table 11-5: Manifestations of Disseminated Candidiasis

- Fever unresponsive to broad-spectrum antimicrobials, frequently the only marker of infection, especially if the patient has:
  - Prolonged intravenous catheterization
  - History of several major risk factors
- Possibly associated with multiorgan infection
- Physical examination is remarkable for the following:
  - Macronodular skin lesions (~10%-20%)
  - Candidal endophthalmitis (~10%-20%)
- Occasionally, septic shock (hypotension, tachycardia, tachypnea)
- Multiorgan dysfunction, depending on the site affected

some of the non-*albicans Candida* species. When candidemia is diagnosed, a general physical examination rarely reveals clinical signs of dissemination, but a thorough examination, especially a dilated funduscopic examination, is mandatory.

Occasionally, blood cultures obtained via central catheters may indicate contamination. Nevertheless, febrile patients with a single positive blood culture for *Candida* species should always initially be considered to have a proven infection. Given the low sensitivity of blood cultures, as well as the lack of a test for the diagnosis of invasive candidiasis, detection of hematogenous dissemination remains poor.

The crude mortality rate reported in patients with candidemia ranges from 40% to 60%, with an attributable mortality of 38%, which exceeds that of most bacteremias.

McNeil et al reported a 50% reduction in national mortality rates for invasive candidiasis since 1989 after a steady increase in mortality in the previous decades, reaching 0.62 death/100,000 population. The decrease in mortality, despite increased invasive disease, may be related to increased awareness, earlier diagnosis, and increased therapeutic options, primarily fluconazole.

Ocular Candidiasis

Candida organisms gain access to the eye by one of two routes: direct inoculation during eye surgery or trauma, or via hematogenous spread (endogenous). Any eye structure may be involved, including the conjunctiva, cornea, lens, ciliary body, vitreous humor, and uveal tract. One or both eyes may be involved. Once endophthalmitis occurs, therapy, especially if delayed, is often insufficient to prevent blindness. Given the recent increased incidence of nosocomial candidemia, a parallel increase in endophthalmitis has occurred. Endophthalmitis should raise the suspicion of concomitant, widely disseminated candidiasis. Estimates of the incidence of eye involvement during candidemia have been as high as 37%, but recent studies indicate a reduced rate of <10%. Only half of cases of endophthalmitis have a history or recent episode of candidemia.

Symptoms of chorioretinitis vary, are often absent in patients too ill to complain, and include visual blurring, floaters, scotomata, and blindness. Funduscopic examination reveals white, cotton-ball-like lesions situated in the chorioretinal layer that may rapidly progress to extend into the posterior vitreous. Indirect ophthalmoscopy with pupillary dilation is necessary to achieve complete visualization. For the lesions to be visible, they require the presence of leukocytes; thus, in the presence of neutropenia, the ocular lesions may be absent.

Diagnosis of *Candida* endophthalmitis is usually made on the basis of clinical context and characteristic funduscopic picture. Aspiration of the anterior chamber is rarely diagnostic, while vitrectomy is often helpful.

Cardiac and Endovascular Candidiasis

Candida myocarditis is the result of hematogenous dissemination with formation of microabscesses within the myocardium that are usually detected only on autopsy. Franklin et al reported that 62% of 50 patients with disseminated candidiasis had myocardial involvement at autopsy.

Candida species may reach the pericardium from adjacent endocarditis or myocarditis, but pericardial involvement is most often the result of hematogenous seeding or direct inoculation during cardiac surgery. Pericarditis is purulent in nature, resembles bacterial infection, and may be complicated by constrictive pericarditis. Successful therapy requires pericardiectomy in addition to antifungal agents. Medical therapy alone is associated with very poor prognosis.

11

Candida *Endocarditis*

The advent of prosthetic cardiac valve surgery and the increase in IV drug abuse have resulted in a dramatic increase in the incidence of *Candida* endocarditis, which previously had been rare. Fungal endocarditis is responsible for <10% of all cases of infective endocarditis. The recent increase in non-*albicans Candida* endocarditis reflects the changing epidemiology of nosocomial candidemia, although it would appear that *C parapsilosis* has a unique affinity for prosthetic valvular surfaces. Another major factor in the epidemiology of *Candida* endocarditis is the recent acceptance by clinicians that all candidemia episodes should be treated.

The pathogenesis of *Candida* endocarditis is complex, but several risk factors have been confirmed. *Candida* organisms rarely adhere to and colonize normal valvular endothelium, but several important predisposing factors have been identified (Table 11-6). *Candida* endocarditis is rare in granulocytopenia, probably because of the short duration of undiagnosed candidemia and universal aggressive therapy. However, it is possible that the accompanying thrombocytopenia may also prevent vegetation formation.

Postoperative endocarditis, especially following prosthetic valve surgery, remains the most common form of *Candida* endocarditis (>50%). However, a recent review concluded that cardiac valve surgery was a decreased risk factor for *Candida* endocarditis. Most episodes occur within 2 months, although endocarditis does occur much later (>12 months). Specific risk factors for prosthetic valve endocarditis include complicated surgery, antibiotics, prolonged postoperative use of catheters, and candidemia, even if transient. Non-*albicans Candida* species are increasingly responsible for prosthetic valve endocarditis, especially *C parapsilosis*. Damaged endocardium and prosthetic material, especially suture lines, serve as foci for *Candida* adherence. Rarely, homografts and heterografts are contaminated before insertion occurs. In addition, pacemaker endocarditis from *Candida* has occurred.

Clinical findings and complications in *Candida* endocarditis are similar to those seen in bacterial endocarditis, with the exceptions of increased frequency of large vegetations and large emboli to major vessels. Aortic and mitral valve involvement are the most common. All the classic findings of bacterial endocarditis have been reported in *Candida* endocarditis, including Osler's nodes, Janeway lesions, splinter hemorrhages, splenomegaly, hematuria, and embolic manifestations. The higher incidence of embolization is frequently manifested as focal and global neurologic deficits. Some studies have found a reduced incidence of cardiac failure, charging heart murmurs, and splenomegaly. Prosthetic valve endocarditis may recur several years after a putative cure with medical therapy, so long-term follow-up is necessary.

Table 11-6: Risk Factors for *Candida* Endocarditis

- Intravenous use of heroin; infection is frequently caused by *Candida parapsilosis*
- Chemotherapy
- Prosthetic valves (~50%)
- Prolonged use of central venous catheters
- Underlying valvular disease
- Preexisting bacterial endocarditis (*C parapsilosis* infection may be superimposed on bacterial endocarditis)
- Immunocompromised host

Most patients with *Candida* endocarditis have positive blood cultures. Improved diagnosis is the result of greater awareness of the significance of candidemia, newer blood culture techniques, and echocardiography. Accordingly, increased preoperative diagnosis has occurred in the last decade. Although not specific for microorganisms, transthoracic and transesophageal echocardiography have made an enormous contribution to avoiding delay in diagnosis. Visualizing large vegetations via echocardiogram in patients with negative blood culture is strong circumstantial evidence of *Candida* endocarditis. Mycologic examination should be performed on all surgically removed emboli.

Candida endocarditis mortality remains high. Before cardiac surgery was available, mortality exceeded 90%. With combined treatment using surgery and aggressive antifungal therapy, mortality rates of ~45% are now typical.

Noncardiac Endovascular Candida *Infections*

The increased incidence of nosocomial candidemia has resulted in the inevitable increase of endovascular infections. Phlebitis due to *Candida* species is common and often associated with subcutaneous catheters. Delay in treatment often results in extensive vascular thrombosis and suppuration. Prolonged candidemia, despite adequate antifungal treatment, is not uncommon. Venous thrombi, even after removal of responsible catheters, impair drug penetration and contain persistent microabscesses, with resultant prolonged candidemia. Surgical excision of thrombi is often required in addition to prolonged antifungal therapy. Complications include superior vena cava obstruction, tricuspid valve endocarditis, right-sided mural endocarditis, and pulmonary vein thrombosis.

Arterial involvement may also occur as a result of candidemia by seeding prosthetic aortic and other large arterial grafts. In addition to pain, fever, and signs of systemic infection, the mycotic aneurysm may rupture, resulting in catastrophic hemorrhage or in large vessel occlusion. *Candida* mycotic aneurysms have been reported in the cerebral circulation, in pulmonary arteries (following use of a Swan-Ganz catheter), in the iliac vessels of IV drug users, and in dialysis shunts.

Chronic Systemic Candidiasis

Hepatosplenic candidiasis (HSC) is a chronic form of disseminated candidiasis that develops as a complication of invasive candidiasis during granulocytopenia. Many now prefer the term chronic systemic candidiasis because other organs (eyes, skin, soft tissue) may be involved. In the last 2 decades, reports of HSC have increased, probably as a result of improved diagnostic imaging and increased rates of candidemia. Candidemia, although frequently secondary to intravascular catheter infection, generally follows *Candida* colonization of the gut, together with disruption of the GI mucosa. This results in invasion of the lamina propria by *Candida* organisms that reach the submucosal blood vessels that drain into the portal venous system and into the liver, where focal lesions are established.

Thus, many patients with chronic systemic candidiasis have no history of documented candidemia. As patients recover from neutropenia, the lesions that were established during the neutropenic phase become more prominent, especially in the liver, spleen, and kidneys.

Clinically, most patients have a history of a hematologic cancer, cytotoxic chemotherapy, or recent recovery from neutropenia, during which time they were febrile and received antibacterial therapy (Table 11-7). Upon recovery from neutropenia, symptoms of antibiotic-resistant fever and abdominal pain begin and worsen as the neutrophils infiltrate foci of *Candida* in the liver and spleen. Serum alkaline phosphatase increases, paralleling the increase in leukocytes, although hepatic transaminases are not commonly elevated.

Lesions of HSC may be detected by imaging techniques such as CT scan, ultrasonography, and magnetic resonance imaging (Table 11-8). The characteristic 'bull's-eye' lesions seen on ultrasound and/or CT are not detectable until neutrophil recovery. However, the lesions are not specific for HSC. As they resolve during therapy, they may either disappear completely or calcify. Ultrasonography appears to be less sensitive but possibly more specific than CT scanning in demonstrating the 'target lesions.' Diagnosis is confirmed by histopathologic examination and culture of hepatic tissue obtained by either percutaneous biopsy or laparoscopy. The appearance of hyphae in a granulomatous lesion is itself not specific for *Candida* and may be caused by other fungi such as *Trichosporon*, *Fusarium*, and *Aspergillus* species. Additionally, metastatic tumors may simulate the appearance of HSC.

Diagnosis

Laboratory Studies

For diagnosis of invasive candidiasis, findings from laboratory studies are nonspecific and lack sensitivity. Clinicians are required to act definitively based on a high

Table 11-7: Manifestations of Chronic Systemic Candidiasis (hepatosplenic candidiasis)

- Fever unresponsive to broad-spectrum antimicrobials
- Right upper quadrant pain
- Nausea and vomiting
- Abdominal pain and distention
- Jaundice (rare)
- Physical examination includes the following:
  - Right upper quadrant tenderness
  - Hepatosplenomegaly (<40%)

index of suspicion. In the past, many patients with life-threatening candidiasis died without receiving antifungal therapy. For therapy to be effective, clinicians must provide it early, frequently, and empirically in patients who are febrile and at risk.

Wet mount smears use scrapings or smears from skin, nails, or oral or vaginal mucosa examined under the microscope to identify hyphae, pseudohyphae, or budding yeast cells.

Potassium hydroxide smear, Gram stain, or methylene blue stain may be used to directly demonstrate fungal cells.

In candidemia and disseminated candidiasis, blood cultures are helpful, but they are positive in only 40% to 60% of cases of disseminated disease. Urinalysis may be helpful and may be indicative of colonization or renal candidiasis. Non-culture-based diagnostic assays are not available in the United States.

Cultures of nonsterile sites, although not useful in establishing a diagnosis, may demonstrate high degrees of

Table 11-8: Imaging Studies Useful in Establishing a Diagnosis of Candidiasis

- Ultrasound may be useful in diagnosing hepatosplenic abscess. The classic 'bull's-eye' or target lesions are seen in the liver and spleen. It can also be useful in demonstrating:
  - Echogenic foci with degrees of shadowing
  - Intra-abdominal abscess formation
  - Cholelithiasis
  - Renal abscess
  - Renal fungus balls
- Computed tomography scan with contrast enhancement may be useful for diagnosing the following:
  - Hepatosplenic candidiasis
  - Intra-abdominal abscess or peritonitis
  - Renal abscess

candidal colonization. This may be useful in initiating antifungal therapy in patients with fever that is unresponsive to broad-spectrum antimicrobials. Therefore, appropriate interpretation is required. Positive blood cultures and cultures from other sterile sites are highly suspicious. Positive results from these sites should always be considered significant and evidence of infection.

Species identification of *Candida* is critically important because of the increase in non-*albicans Candida* species. CHROMagar *Candida* media allows for the presumptive identification of several *Candida* species by using color reactions in specialized media that demonstrate different colony colors. Several biochemical assays can be used to identify the different *Candida* species with more accuracy. These assays evaluate the assimilation of a number of carbon substrates and generate profiles used in the identification of different fungal species. Recently, a new sensitive commercial test for *Candida* diagnosis has been introduced via Fungitell assay which measures the amount of β-D-glucan released from the fungal cell wall. Sensitivity for *Candida* infections was 81.3%. The test often provides a positive rest day before clinical signs and symptoms appear, allowing earlier initiation of therapy.

Molecular assays such as polymerase chain reaction tests and DNA probes are still under development and in the early investigational phases, but they appear promising.

The NCCLS microbroth dilution methodology has standardized antifungal susceptibility testing for *Candida* species (Tables 11-9, 11-10, and 11-11). Although not used as a standard of care, it may be helpful in guiding difficult therapeutic decisions. Most of the difficult decisions involve antifungal therapy for refractory oral or esophageal candidiasis in patients with advanced HIV.

Management

Treatment of *Candida* infections varies considerably and is based on the anatomic location of the infection, the patient's underlying disease and immune status, the patient's risk factors for infection, the specific species of *Candida* responsible for infection, and, in some cases, the susceptibility of the strain to antifungal drugs (Table 11-12). In 2009, the Infectious Diseases Society of America published new practice guidelines for the treatment of candidiasis.

Azoles have been the mainstay of therapy for the past 10 to 15 years, including topical and systemic agents. Polyenes include amphotericin B, liposomal amphotericin B formulations, and topical nystatin (Mycostatin®). The echinocandin class of antifungals with their excellent fungicidal activity against *Candida* species have recently gained rapid acceptance in the management of candidal infections.

The primary difference between the newer treatment guidelines and the prior guidelines has to do with the up-front use of echinocandins in patients with candidemia and suspected candidiasis who have moderate to severe infections, in patients with infections due to *C glabrata* and *C krusei*, and in patients with a history of azole exposure.

Cutaneous Candidiasis

Most localized, cutaneous candidiasis infections can be treated with topical antifungal agents, such as clotrimazole (Lotrimin®, Mycelex-G®), econazole (Spectazole®), ciclopirox (Loprox®), miconazole (Monistat®, Micatin®), ketoconazole (Nizoral®), and nystatin. If the infection is a paronychia, the most important aspect of the therapy is drainage of the abscess, followed by oral antifungal therapy with either fluconazole or itraconazole (Sporanox®). In cases of extensive cutaneous infections, infections in immunocompromised patients, folliculitis, or onychomycosis, systemic antifungal therapy is recommended. For *Candida* onychomycosis, oral itraconazole appears to be the most efficacious. Two treatment regimens are available: a single daily dose of itraconazole taken for 3 to 6 months or a pulsed-dose regimen that requires a slightly higher dose daily for 7 days, followed by 3 weeks off therapy. The cycle is repeated every month for 3 to 6 months.

Gastrointestinal Candidiasis

OPC may be treated with topical antifungal agents (nystatin, clotrimazole, amphotericin B oral suspension) or with systemic oral azoles (fluconazole, itraconazole) (Table 11-13).

Candida esophagitis requires systemic therapy, usually with fluconazole or itraconazole for at least 14 to 21 days. Parenteral therapy with fluconazole may be required initially if the patient is unable to take oral medications. Daily suppressive antifungal therapy with fluconazole 100 to 200

Table 11-9: In Vitro Susceptibility of *Candida* Species to Azole Antifungal Agents*

Candida Species	Fluconazole (MIC_{50})
C albicans	1
C tropicalis	1
C glabrata	16
C parapsilosis	1
C krusei	64
C lusitaniae	2

MIC_{50} = median minimum inhibitory concentration (μg/mL)

*Based on 2,047 blood culture isolates collected from January 1997 through December 2000. Susceptibilities were calculated

mg/d is effective in preventing recurrent episodes, but it should only be used if the recurrences become frequent or are associated with malnutrition from poor oral intake and wasting syndrome. In patients with advanced AIDS and profound immunodeficiency, recurrent EC caused by azole-resistant *C albicans* or *C glabrata* can be effectively treated with either voriconazole (Vfend®), caspofungin (Cancidas®), or anidulafungin (Eraxis™).

Genital Tract Candidiasis

Vulvovaginal candidiasis can be managed with either topical antifungal agents or single-dose oral fluconazole for uncomplicated infections (Table 11-14). Single-dose (150 mg) oral fluconazole has been shown to have clinical and microbiologic efficacy as good as that of topical antifungal agents for the treatment of VVC.

Voriconazole (MIC_{50})	Itraconazole (MIC_{50})	Posaconazole (MIC_{50})
0.06	0.5	0.13
2	1	1
0.5	0.25	1
0.06	0.12	0.13
1	0.5	0.5
0.06	0.25	0.13

on the basis of NCCLS methodology. Pfaller et al, *J Clin Microbiol* 2002;40:852-856.

A small percentage of women (<5%) suffer from chronic recurrent VVC infections, which often require chronic or prophylactic oral azole therapy for control. In women who suffer from recurrent attacks, the standard recommended regimen is fluconazole at a dose of 150 mg every third day for 3 doses, followed by weekly fluconazole at a dose of 150 mg for 6 months. This regimen prevents recurrent infections in more than 90% of women.

Urinary Tract Candidiasis—Candiduria

Asymptomatic candiduria in urinary catheterized patients is extremely common and generally reflects yeast colonization of the catheter and lower urinary tract and, hence, antifungal therapy is not indicated. Symptomatic candiduria reflects deep tissue on parenchymal invasion and results in organ-specific as well as constitutional symptoms

Table 11-10: In Vitro Susceptibility of *Candida* Species to Other Antifungal Agents*

Candida Species	Amphotericin B** (MIC_{50})	Flucytosine** (MIC_{50})
C albicans	0.5	≤0.25
C tropicalis	0.25	≤0.25
C glabrata	0.5	≤0.25
C parapsilosis	0.25	≤0.25
C krusei	0.25	16
C lusitaniae	≥1	≤0.25

MIC_{50} = median minimum inhibitory concentration (µg/mL)

*Susceptibilities were calculated on the basis of NCCLS methodology.

**Pfaller et al, *J Clin Microbiol* 2002;40:852-856.

(eg, fever, frequency, dysuria [lower urinary tract] and fever, renal angle pain, nausea, vomiting, and even sepsis [pyelonephritis]). While amphotericin B IV has been the mainstay of indicated therapy, accompanying drug nephrotoxicity limits its use. Fluconazole, 400 mg/d, uniquely achieving high urinary concentrations, has emerged as the drug of first choice with small dose adjustments required for coexistent renal insufficiency. None of the other azoles, including voriconazole, are excreted in urine. Similarly, the echinocandins achieve minimal subtherapeutic urine concentrations. A useful agent for eradicating non-*albicans* candidemia, especially *C glabrata,* is oral flucytosine in the absence of renal failure. Deep tissue invasion of kidneys or bladder can be treated by all the systemically active antifungals.

Caspofungin† (MIC_{50})	Micafungin† (MIC_{50})	Anidulafungin† (MIC_{50})
0.5	0.03	0.03
1	0.06	0.06
2	0.06	0.06
2	2	2
2	0.25	0.13
1	1	0.25

† Rex JH: Antifungal susceptibility survey of 2,000 bloodstream *Candida* isolates from the United States. 39th Meeting of the Infectious Diseases Society of America; October 25-28, 2001; San Francisco, CA. Abstract 642.

Candidemia and Acute Disseminated Candidiasis

Candidemia requires treatment in all patients (Figure 11-5). It is related to the presence of an intravascular catheter in up to 80% of non-neutropenic patients. Removal of intravascular catheters appears to shorten the duration of candidemia and has been associated with reduced mortality. Some patients have even been cured by catheter removal alone. However, even transient episodes of candidemia can be associated with subsequent hematogenous spread that causes endophthalmitis or osteomyelitis. Thus, all episodes of candidemia merit antifungal therapy. A dilated retinal examination is important in all candidemic patients.

While amphotericin B has been the standard approach, two prospective randomized trials and two retrospective reviews compared amphotericin B with fluconazole.

Table 11-11: Management of Candidemia and Disseminated Candidiasis

- **For *C albicans, C parapsilosis, C tropicalis, C lusitaniae, C dubliniensis***
  - Fluconazole 800 mg x 1 dose, followed by 400 mg/d IV or PO
  - Caspofungin (Cancidas®) 70 mg x 1 dose, followed by 50 mg q.d. IV
  - Anidulafungin (Eraxis™) 200 mg x 1 dose, followed by 100 mg/d IV
  - Micafungin (Mycamine®) 100 mg/d IV
- **For *C glabrata***
  - (Select therapy on the basis of MICs)
  - Caspofungin 70 mg x 1 dose, followed by 50 mg/d IV
  - Anidulafungin 200 mg x 1 dose, followed by 100 mg/d IV
  - Micafungin (Mycamine®) 100 mg/d IV
  - Voriconazole 6 mg/kg q 12 h x 2, followed by 3 mg/kg q 12 h
  - Amphotericin B 0.7-1.0 mg/kg/d
  - Fluconazole 800 mg/d
- **For *C krusei***
  - Caspofungin 70 mg x 1 d, 50 mg/d
  - Anidulafungin 200 mg x 1 dose, followed by 100 mg/d IV
  - Micafungin (Mycamine®) 100 mg/d IV
  - Voriconazole 6 mg/kg q 12 h x 2, followed by 3 mg/kg q 12 h

Table 11-12: Interpretive Breakpoints for *Candida* Species

		Minimum Inhibitory Concentration, µg/mL	
Drug	**S**	**S-DD or I**	**R**
Fluconazole	≤8	S-DD, 16-32	>32
Itraconazole	≤0.125	S-DD, 0.25-0.5	>0.5
Flucytosine	≤4	I, 8-16	>16
Voriconazole	≤1		2>4

S = susceptible; R = resistant
S-DD = susceptible-dose dependent; I = intermediate

The studies demonstrated that amphotericin B at 0.5 to 0.6 mg/kg/d and fluconazole at 400 mg/d are equivalent as effective therapy of candidemia in non-neutropenic patients (Table 11-15). In all four studies, most isolates were *C albicans*. The strength of the data is less reassuring for non-*albicans Candida* species, but similar trends hold. Non-*albicans Candida* species, especially *C glabrata*, have higher fluconazole minimum inhibitory concentrations, so higher antifungal doses may be required for optimal outcome. Anidulafungin (Eraxis®), caspofungin (Cancidas®), and micafungin (Mycamine®) have also been proven effective in candidemia and invasive candidiasis. The broad spectrum anti-*Candida* activity of echinocandins, together with rapid fungicidal action, and ease of use, make the echinocandin class highly suitable for therapy, especially given their safety profile and easy use in renal failure and liver disease. In a recent study, anidulafungin (Eraxis™) was found to be superior to fluconazole in candidemia patients. In another study, voriconazole was shown to be equivalent

Table 11-13: Oropharyngeal and Esophageal Candidiasis Treatment Options

Treatment Options	Dosing Guidelines
Nystatin (Mycostatin®) Pastilles or lozenge	200,000 U q.i.d. x 7-14 d
Suspension	500,000 U by swish and swallow q.i.d. x 7-14 d
Vaginal tablets	100,000 U dissolve 1 tab t.i.d.
Clotrimazole	Suck on 1 troche 5 x d x 7-14 d
Fluconazole Oral suspension or oral tablet	100 mg/d x 7-14 d (up to 21 d for esophagitis); loading dose of 200 mg for severe OPC and esophagitis
Itraconazole	
Solution	200 mg (20 mL) q.d. by swish and swallow x 7-14 d (up to 21 d for esophagitis)
Capsules	200 mg/d (with food) x 2-4 wk
Ketoconazole	200-400 mg/d x 7-14 d (up to 21 d for esophagitis)

q.i.d. = four times daily; t.i.d. = three times daily;
b.i.d. = twice daily; q.d. = once daily;
OPC = oropharyngeal candidiasis

to a strategy of amphotericin B followed by fluconazole. Accordingly, a number of potent antifungal agents can be empirically selected in the initial therapy for candidemia. In two recent studies, micafungin was shown to be as good

Patient/Prescribing Issues

Unpleasant taste; may cause nausea and gastrointestinal disturbances.

Not recommended for esophagitis.

More palatable than nystatin but contains dextrose, which may promote dental caries; not recommended for esophagitis.

Superior to nystatin, clotrimazole, ketoconazole. High doses (up to 800 mg/d) can be used in difficult cases. Success has been obtained even in cases of in vitro resistance.

11

Limited bioavailability; absorption improved if taken with fatty meal; efficacy of capsules is thought to be equal to that of ketoconazole. Solution has been tested only among HIV patients but is much better absorbed and has shown efficacy equivalent to that of fluconazole.

Limited bioavailability; requires acidic environment for best absorption; liver toxicity; less efficacious than fluconazole and itraconazole and less frequently used.

(continued on next page)

as AmBisome® and caspofungin for candidemia and disseminated candidiasis.

Until recently, many clinicians treated *C glabrata* fungemia with intravenous (IV) fluconazole 800 mg/d (12

Table 11-13: Oropharyngeal and Esophageal Candidiasis Treatment Options *(continued)*

Treatment Options	Dosing Guidelines
Amphotericin B	
Suspension	1 mg/mL 1 mL swish and swallow q.i.d.
Lozenge	100 mg q.i.d.
Tablet	10 mg q.i.d.
Parenteral	0.4-0.6 mg/kg/d
Echinocandins	
Anidulafungin (Eraxis™)	100 mg IV x 1 followed by 50 mg/d
Caspofungin (Cancidas®)	70 mg IV x 1 followed by 50 mg/d
Micafungin (Mycamine®)	150 mg/d IV

q.i.d. = four times daily; t.i.d. = three times daily; b.i.d. = twice daily; q.d. = once daily; OPC = oropharyngeal candidiasis

mg/kg) in adults with normal renal function. The results of only one noncomparative study suggest that 800 mg/d may produce a better response rate than 400 mg/d for *C albicans* fungemia. Choosing between initial polyene, triazoles, or echinocandin is somewhat arbitrary. However, in unstable, critically ill patients with little margin for error, in patients previously exposed to fluconazole, or in patients infected with either *C glabrata* or *C krusei*, initiating treatment with amphotericin B or an echinocandin is recommended. Additionally, a study by the Mycoses Study Group suggests

Patient/Prescribing Issues

Agent considered second-line option; reserved for severe cases and documented failures to azoles; parenteral dosing necessary for esophagitis.

Agents are second-line options; parenteral dosing only.

11

a possible advantage in initiating treatment with a combination of fluconazole and amphotericin B. Combinations of either fluconazole or amphotericin B with flucytosine (Ancobon®) at 100 to 150 mg/kg/d may be useful in some patients, but the precise role of this combination is unclear. The required duration of antifungal therapy is undetermined, but therapy is usually continued for about 2 weeks after the last positive blood culture. With this approach, the rate of subsequent recurrent infection at a hematogenously seeded site is about 1%.

Table 11-14: Azole Therapy for Vaginal Candidiasis

Drug	Formulation	Dosage
Butoconazole (Femstat 3®, Gynazole-1®)	2% cream	5 g x 3 d single dose
Clotrimazole	1% cream	5 g x 7-14 d
	10% cream	5 g single application
	100-mg vaginal tablet	1 tablet x 7 d
	100-mg vaginal tablet	2 tablets x 3 d
	500-mg vaginal tablet	1 tablet once
Miconazole	2% cream	5 g x 7 d
(Femizol-M®, Monistat®)	100-mg vaginal suppository	1 suppository x 7 d
	200-mg vaginal suppository	1 suppository x 3 d
	1200-mg vaginal suppository	1 suppository once

Although the gut has been implicated as the source of candidemia in non-neutropenic patients, it appears likely that the GI tract is the most common source of candidemia in neutropenic patients. In these patients, removal of intravenous catheters may still be important. One notable exception is *C parapsilosis* fungemia, which is highly associated with intravascular catheters in cancer patients. Recovery of marrow function is critical, and no therapeutic approach is consistently successful in the face of persistent leukopenia. For candidemia in neutropenic patients, the current recommendation is either an echinocandin (anidu-

Drug	Formulation	Dosage
Econazole	150-mg vaginal tablet	1 tablet x 3 d
Fenticonazole	2% cream	5 g x 7 d
Tioconazole	2% cream	5 g x 3 d
(Vagistat-1®)	6.5% cream	5 g single dose
Terconazole	0.4% cream	5 g x 7 d
(Terazol® 3,	0.8% cream	5 g x 3 d
Terazol® 7)	80-mg vaginal suppository	80 mg x 3 d
Fluconazole	Oral tablet	150 mg single dose
Ketoconazole	200-mg tablet	400 mg x 5 d
Itraconazole	100-mg tablet	200 mg x 3 d

lafungin, caspofungin, micafungin) or a lipid amphotericin B preparation 3-5 mg/kg/d IV. In patients who are stable and not critical, use either fluconazole 12 mg/kg/d x 1 dose, followed by 6 mg/kg/day, or voriconazole 6 mg/kg b.i.d x 1 day, followed by 4 mg/kg b.i.d. However, for infections due to *C glabrata* or *C krusei*, an echinocandin is the recommended antifungal. The use of flucytosine is limited because of its potential for marrow suppression and the lack of a readily available IV formulation.

Patients may develop candidemia while already on antifungal therapy, including prophylactic antifungals.

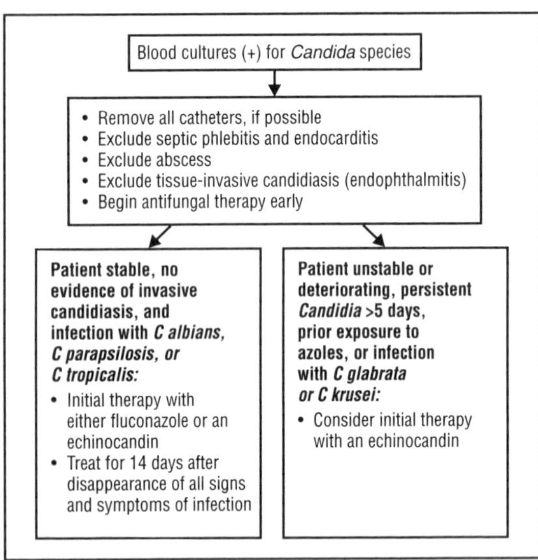

Figure 11-5: Management algorithm for hematogenous candidiasis.

Such breakthrough candidemia may be the result of an infected, unremoved intravascular catheter. In cancer patients, breakthrough candidemia has been associated with a higher mortality and has occurred more often during an ICU stay, during prolonged neutropenia, and with the use of corticosteroids. In this setting, immunosuppression should be reduced and factors that might alter antifungal drug delivery or clearance excluded. Intravenous catheters should be changed and the possibility of drug resistance considered, especially since non-*albicans Candida* species are frequently responsible. Antifungal susceptibility tests should be performed. Therapy should be changed to an antifungal of a different class.

Table 11-15: First-Line Therapy for Candidemia and Invasive Candidiasis

Polyenes

- Amphotericin B deoxycholate (Fungizone®) 0.5-0.7 mg/kg/d
- Liposomal amphotericin B (AmBisome®) 3-5 mg/kg/d
- Lipid complex amphotericin B (Abelcet®) 3-5 mg/kg/d

Azoles

- Fluconazole IV 400-800 mg/d
- Voriconazole (Vfend®) IV 6 mg followed by 3 mg/kg b.i.d.

Echinocandins

- Caspofungin (Cancidas®) IV 70 mg and 50 mg/d
- Micafungin (Mycamine®) IV 100 mg/d, pending FDA approval
- Anidulafungin (Eraxis™) IV 200 mg x 1 dose, followed by 100 mg/d

Nonsubcutaneous tunnel central intravascular catheters should be removed in non-neutropenic patients with candidemia. A suspect catheter should not be replaced over a guide wire if this procedure can be avoided. In contrast, central tunneled catheters in febrile neutropenic patients do not require mandatory removal because alternate vascular access sites are less available, removal is more difficult, and, most importantly, such catheters are less likely to be the source of candidemia, although they may become infected secondarily to blood stream infection. Occasionally, these valuable access sites can be salvaged using the controversial antibiotic lock method with amphotericin B, but results are unpredictable. The importance of a positive catheter tip is similarly controversial. In afebrile patients at low risk of candidemia, antifungal treatment does not appear to be indicated. On the other hand, in a high-risk patient with unexplained antibiotic-resistant fever, the finding of a positive catheter tip often results in initiation of empirical antifungal therapy.

Chronic Disseminated Candidiasis

Therapy of chronic disseminated candidiasis or HSC traditionally consists of prolonged therapy with fluconazole 800 mg x 1 dose, followed by 400 mg/d in stable patients. In severely ill patients, either lipid amphotericin B 3-5 mg/kg/d or amphotericin B deoxycholate 0.7-1.0 mg/kg/d IV is recommended. Recently, echinocandins for 2 weeks, followed by fluconazole, has also been shown to be successful. If the lesions have stabilized, the patient is clinically improved, and antifungal therapy is continued, antineoplastic therapies (including those that induce neutropenia) may be continued. The duration of antifungal therapy is determined by imaging studies of the liver and spleen.

Selecting Antifungals

Fluconazole has been the drug of choice in the routine management of many candidemia and disseminated candidiasis infections. Studies conducted by the Mycoses Study Group have demonstrated that fluconazole at a dose of 400 mg/d is as effective as amphotericin B. In addition, fluconazole has several advantages, including lower nephrotoxicity (<2%) and ease of use because of its high degree of oral bioavailability. Thus, once the GI tract is functional, the parenteral dose may be switched to the oral formulation with the same efficacy.

The standard recommended dose for most *Candida* infections is fluconazole 800 mg as the loading dose, followed by fluconazole at a dose of 400 mg/d (Table 11-13). This treatment regimen can be used for infections caused by *C albicans*, *C tropicalis*, *C parapsilosis*, *Candida kefyr*, *Candida dubliniensis*, *C lusitaniae*, and *C guilliermondii*.

The echinocandins (caspofungin, micafungin, and anidulafungin) have gained wide acceptance in the management of candidemia and invasive candidiasis. The echinocandins have recently become drugs of choice for the management of these infections.

Although amphotericin B has been the standard in systemic fungal infections for 30 years despite a high adverse effect profile, it is now an alternative in most cases of candidemia or disseminated candidiasis. The standard dose for amphotericin B is 0.7 to 1.0 mg/kg/d to achieve a minimum of 500 to 1000 mg total dose.

Certain situations involving several *Candida* species require special mention. Infections due to *C glabrata*, because of its intrinsic lower susceptibility to all antifungals, and the incidence of fluconazole resistance, require the knowledge of the antifungal activity of antifungals against several of the *Candida* species. In infections due to *C glabrata*, the initial drugs of choice are the echinocandins (anidulafungin, caspofungin, micafungin). Other reasonable alternatives include voriconazole 4 mg/kg b.i.d., lipid amphotericin B 3-5 mg/kg/d, or amphotericin B deoxycholate 1 mg/kg/d. Also important are infections due to *C krusei* because of its intrinsic resistance to ketoconazole, fluconazole, or itraconazole. The initial drugs of choice are also the echinocandins, voriconazole 4 mg/kg b.i.d, lipid amphotericin B 3-5 mg/kg/d, or amphotericin B deoxycholate 1 mg/kg/d. Caspofungin, micafungin, and anidulafungin are FDA approved for use in the treatment of systemic *Candida* infections, although *C parapsilosis* has shown reduced susceptibility to these agents. Voriconazole at 3 mg/kg q 12 h IV or 200 mg orally q 12 h may also be a broad-spectrum, first-line alternative. Infections caused by *C lusitaniae* or *C guilliermondii* require the use of fluconazole or caspofungin because these isolates frequently are intrinsically resistant to amphotericin B or develop resistance to amphotericin B in vivo while the patient is on therapy.

The optimum dosage and duration of therapy for various types of deep candidal infection have not been definitively determined. However, therapy for candidemia should be continued for at least 2 weeks after the last positive blood culture and after signs and symptoms of infection have resolved. Disseminated candidiasis with end-organ involvement requires an individualized approach. Thus, invasive candidiasis involving localized structures, such as *Candida* osteomyelitis, arthritis, endocarditis, pericarditis, and meningitis, requires prolonged antifungal therapy for at least 4 to 6 weeks.

A critical component in the management of candidemia and disseminated candidiasis is the removal of the focus of infection, such as IV and Foley catheters. In addition, starting antifungal therapy as early as possible is necessary, as soon as adequate cultures are obtained.

The combination of amphotericin B and flucytosine has been recommended in several special situations, particularly for patients who are immunocompromised with *Candida* endophthalmitis and *Candida* meningitis. Flucytosine appears to interact synergistically with amphotericin B in animal models. Lipid preparations of amphotericin B have also been used successfully. Caspofungin acetate has also been demonstrated to be as good as, or superior to, amphotericin B, without the nephrotoxicity and may emerge as a drug of choice for candidemia.

Prevention

Prophylaxis of Candidiasis in Transplant Patients

Invasive candidal infections are a concern in this high-risk group. Institutions with recipients of solid-organ and bone marrow transplants usually consider prophylaxis with fluconazole for the prevention of candidiasis. Fluconazole is generally started 1 day before neutropenia, and some investigators support its use for 75 to 100 days after bone marrow transplantation. In liver transplants, short-term fluconazole prophylaxis is indicated in selected high-risk patients.

Prophylaxis of Superficial Candidiasis in HIV-positive Patients

There is little support for primary or secondary prevention of OPC, esophageal candidiasis, or vaginal candidiasis in HIV-positive patients. Concern about the potential development of resistance or colonization by resistant species or strains of *Candida* does exist. Prophylaxis may be indicated in a select group of patients with recurrent symptomatic candidiasis only.

Empiric Anti-*Candida* Treatment

Empiric use of antifungal agents in febrile patients in ICUs is widespread without supporting data. Given the existing difficulties in diagnosing invasive candidiasis, it appears reasonable to recommend empiric antifungal therapy in selected febrile, high-risk patients with persistent antibiotic-resistant fever. Echinocandins, with their broad-spectrum, excellent anticandidal activity, low incidence of adverse events, and ease of use, are preferable options as initial antifungal therapy in these types of patients. This is especially true in patients who are severely ill, who are hemodynamically unstable, who are in septic shock from *Candida* species, who are infected with an unknown *Candida* species, or who have had previous exposure to azole antifungals. The use of empiric antifungals in low-risk patients is not justified.

Suggested Readings

Calderone RA: *Candida and Candidiasis*. Washington, DC: ASM Press, 2001.

Edwards, JE. Candida species. In: Mandell GL, Bennett JE, Dolin R, eds. *Principles and Practice of Infectious Diseases*, 5th ed. New York, NY, Churchill Livingstone, 2000, pp 2656-2674.

Eggimann P, Garbino J, Pittet D: Management of *Candida* species infections in critically ill patients. *Lancet Infect Dis* 2003;3: 772-785.

Golan Y, Wolf MP, Pauker SG, et al: Empirical anti-Candida therapy among selected patients in the intensive care unit: a cost-effectiveness analysis. *Ann Intern Med* 2005;143:857-869.

Kullberg BJ, Sobel JD, Ruhnke M, et al: Voriconazole versus a regimen of amphotericin B followed by fluconazole for candidemia in non-neutropenic patients: a randomized non-inferiority trial. *Lancet* 2005 28;366:1435-1442.

Mora-Duarte J, Betts R, Rotstein C, et al: Caspofungin Invasive Candidiasis Study Group. Comparison of caspofungin and amphotericin B for invasive candidiasis. *N Engl J Med* 2002;347: 2020-2029.

Pappas PG, Kaufman CA, Andes D, et al: Clinical practice guidelines for the management of candidiasis: 2009 update by the Infectious Diseases Society of America. *Clin Infect Dis* 2009;48(5):503-535.

Pappas PG, Rex JH, Lee J, et al: NIAID Mycoses Study Group. A prospective observational study of candidemia: epidemiology, therapy, and influences on mortality in hospitalized adult and pediatric patients. *Clin Infect Dis* 2003;37:634-643.

Pappas PG, Rex JH, Sobel JD, et al: Infectious Diseases Society of America. Guidelines for treatment of candidiasis. *Clin Infect Dis* 2004;38:161-189.

Pappas PG, Rotstein CM, Betts RF, et al: Micafungin versus caspofungin for treatment of candidemia and other forms of invasive candidiasis. *Clin Infect Dis* 2007;45:883-893.

Reboli AC, Rotstein C, Pappas PG, et al, and the Anidulafungin Study Group: Anidulafugin versus fluconazole for invasive candidiasis. *N Engl J Med* 2007;356:2472-2482.

Zaoutis TE, Argon J, Chu J, et al: The epidemiology and attributable outcomes of candidemia in adults and children hospitalized in the United States: a propensity analysis. *Clin Infect Dis 2005;4: 1232-1239*

Chapter 12

Cryptococcosis

Cryptococcus neoformans is a widespread, pathogenic, encapsulated yeast that causes human diseases ranging from asymptomatic pulmonary colonization to life-threatening meningitis and overwhelming cryptococcemia. Although disease may occur in normal hosts, most patients usually have advanced underlying disorders of the immune system. The dominant underlying predisposing factor is a defect in T-cell immunity. Nevertheless, life-threatening disease can also occur in otherwise-normal hosts. 12

Cryptococcosis is caused by two varieties of *C neoformans*: variety *neoformans* (serotypes A and D) and variety *gattii* (serotypes B and C). The disease caused by variety *neoformans* occurs throughout the world, whereas the disease caused by variety *gattii* has mainly been prevalent in tropical and subtropical areas. The virulence, chronicity, and clinical course of cryptococcosis caused by *C neoformans* var. *gattii* differ from those associated with cryptococcosis caused by *C neoformans* var. *neoformans*. *Cryptococcus neoformans* is an encapsulated yeast 4 to 6 microns in diameter that is definitively diagnosed by a positive culture. The organism grows on modified Sabouraud's dextrose agar and other selective media for fungi, generally within 4 to 7 days after inoculation. Other tests are also useful in establishing a diagnosis of cryptococcal infection. Unlike other nonpathogenic cryptococcal species, *C neoformans* grows well at 37°C.

Cryptococcus neoformans is a basidiomycetous fungus, and its main habitat is the debris around pigeon roosts and soil that is contaminated by decaying pigeon or chicken droppings. Not a part of the normal microbial flora of humans, *C neoformans* is only transiently isolated from individuals with no pathologic features. It is generally accepted that the organism enters the host by the respiratory route in the form of a dehydrated haploid yeast or as basidiospores. After some time in the lung, the organism hematogenously spreads to extrapulmonary tissues, especially the brain. As a result, infected persons usually contract meningoencephalitis. Dissemination may involve other sites, including skin, bone, and the urinary tract.

Virulence factors for this life-threatening pathogen include the polysaccharide capsule, shed products of the organisms, melanin production, mannitol secretion, superoxide dismutase, proteases, and phospholipases. Of these virulence factors, the polysaccharide serves to inhibit phagocytosis by polymorphonuclear leukocytes, monocytes, and macrophages. The effectiveness of many of these cryptococcal virulence factors depends on the status of the host defensive mechanism.

Because the dominant disease manifestation involves infection of the central nervous system (CNS), this chapter concentrates on meningoencephalitis. Cryptococcosis has been identified in 30% of HIV-positive patients in Africa and Southeast Asia but occurs less often in industrialized countries (6% to 10% of HIV-infected patients in the United States have cryptococcosis). *Cryptococcus neoformans* is the most common cause of fungal meningitis worldwide, and it is a common problem among HIV-infected patients. Before the HIV epidemic, most patients with cryptococcosis had underlying disorders associated with cell-mediated immune dysfunction, such as corticosteroid treatment, solid organ transplantation, hematologic malignancies, or sarcoidosis. However, in that time, up to 40% of patients with cryptococcosis had

Table 12-1: Clinical Features of Cryptococcosis

Meningeal Infection	
Fever	60%-90%
Headache	80%-90%
Nausea/vomiting	~50%
Meningism	30%
Altered mental status	20%-30%
Extrameningeal Infection	
Lung	
Bone marrow	
Skin	
Prostate (a cryptic source)	

no underlying disorder associated with immune dysfunction. Selected defects in lymphocyte responsiveness to *C neoformans* have been offered to explain disease occurrence in otherwise-normal hosts. The variety *gattii* is more commonly seen in immunocompetent patients, and its rarity in immunocompromised patients remains unexplained.

Cryptococcal Meningitis

Cryptococcal CNS infection generally manifests as subacute or chronic meningoencephalitis, although individuals may present with acute illness (Table 12-1). The duration of symptoms before admission is often several days to weeks. The most common clinical symptoms are headache (80% to 90%), fever (60% to 90%), nausea or vomiting (50% to 60%), altered mental status (20% to 50%), stiff neck (30% to 50%), cranial nerve palsies (10% to 30%), papilledema (20% to 30%), cerebellar signs (10% to 25%), and seizures (5% to 15%). Patients with

Table 12-2: Cryptococcal Meningitis—Laboratory Parameters

- Cerebrospinal fluid
  - ↑ pressure
  - ↑ minimal white blood cell count
  - ↑ protein
  - Cryptococcal antigen
- Blood culture
- Serum cryptococcal antigen

advanced cryptococcal meningitis with raised intracranial pressure may present with sudden blindness, deafness, or coma. Alterations in the state of consciousness, visual defects, and papilledema occur more frequently in non-immunosuppressed patients than in patients with AIDS. Fever is not always present, and neck stiffness is frequently absent, so it is not usually difficult to distinguish cryptococcal meningitis from other bacterial and viral causes of meningitis. Often, the clinical presentation simulates an encephalopathy; therefore, the differential diagnosis in HIV-infected patients with such symptoms includes toxoplasmosis, primary CNS lymphoma, progressive multifocal leukoencephalopathy, cytomegalovirus disease, and HIV encephalopathy. Laboratory findings include an elevated opening pressure when a spinal tap is performed, with spinal fluid pressures frequently in excess of 250 mm H_2O and occasionally exceeding 500 mm H_2O. Accordingly, measurement of the opening pressure is a crucial step in the investigation of an HIV-infected patient with meningoencephalitis. The cerebrospinal fluid (CSF) protein is elevated in most patients but does not commonly exceed 100 mg/dL; CSF pleocytosis is variable (Table 12-2).

Table 12-3: Indicators of Poor Prognosis

- Altered mental state
- CSF white blood cell count <20 cells/mm^3
- CSF cryptococcal antigen >1:10,000
- Other predictors
  - No prior antiretroviral therapy
  - Visual abnormalities

CSF = cerebrospinal fluid

A striking feature of cryptococcal meningitis is the paucity of cellular response that is predominantly lymphocytic in nature. Hypoglycorrhachia is frequently present. A positive India ink preparation has been found in 75% of HIV-infected patients, compared with 30% of non-HIV-infected patients. Cryptococcal antigen titers are found in the CSF in more than 98% of AIDS patients with cryptococcal meningitis, and the median CSF cryptococcal antigen titer is 1:1,024. There exists a strong correlation between CSF cryptococcal antigen titers and CSF cryptococcal colony-forming unit counts. Serum cryptococcal antigen titers are also positive in more than 98% of AIDS patients with cryptococcal disease, and the titer tends to be even higher in these cases (usually >2,048). Poor-prognosis indicators are listed in Table 12-3.

Although the computed tomography (CT) scan of the head is abnormal in up to 30% of patients with cryptococcal meningitis, the most common abnormality is cortical atrophy. Ventricular enlargement reflecting obstruction or hydrocephalus is uncommon in AIDS patients. Cryptococcomas may present as enhancing abscesses or mass lesions. In general, most physicians advocate CT scanning and/or magnetic resonance imaging before performing lumbar puncture in any HIV-infected patients who present with fever and headache. Intracerebral cryptococcal lesions may occur as gelatinous pseudocysts, granulomas, or mixed forms. Although they can produce symptoms of an expanding intracranial lesion, most intracerebral lesions tend to be asymptomatic. Larger cryptococcomas are more characteristic of infection caused by the variety *gattii*.

In patients with advanced HIV infection, other CNS manifestations are more likely to be present, including positive blood cultures and pulmonary manifestations, such as cough, chest pain, and dyspnea. Radiologic features include nodular or cavitary lesions or asymmetric pulmonary infiltrates (Figure 12-1; see color plate insert). Occasionally, patients may exhibit cutaneous manifestations such as umbilicated papular lesions. Involvement of the urinary tract is also common. Although clinical manifestations are rare, prostatic tissue is considered to be an important reservoir for future cryptococcal reactivation. In Africa, concomitant tuberculous meningitis is frequently present, adding significantly to the morbidity and mortality of cryptococcal meningitis.

Treatment of Cryptococcal Meningitis

Until the mid-1970s, the standard therapy for cryptococcal meningitis was monotherapy with amphotericin B (Amphocin®, Fungizone®). In a classic study, Bennett et al established the superior efficacy of combination therapy with amphotericin B and flucytosine (Ancobon®) for 6 weeks, compared with amphotericin B alone for 10 weeks. In recent years, fluconazole (Diflucan®), which has excellent in vitro and in vivo activity against *C neoformans*, has become widely used for the treatment of cryptococcosis. All subsequent large prospective clinical studies established the importance and value of fluconazole in the management of cryptococcosis; these studies have

Table 12-4: Management of Cryptococcal Meningitis in AIDS

Acute Induction Therapy

- Amphotericin B 0.7 mg/kg + flucytosine 100 mg/kg for a minimum of 2 weeks followed by fluconazole 400 mg/d for 6 weeks

Maintenance Phase for Life in HIV-positive Patients

- Fluconazole 200 mg/d

been exclusively conducted among HIV-infected patients. Similar studies have not been performed in HIV-negative patients, and, therefore, many of the recommendations and current approaches to the management of cryptococcosis in HIV-negative patients are derived from experience with the HIV-positive population.

Before amphotericin B became available, cryptococcal meningitis was considered uniformly fatal. Amphotericin B has been the drug of choice since the late 1950s, with success rates approaching 60%. Successful therapy, however, was limited by nephrotoxicity, electrolyte abnormalities, and infusion-related adverse events. Based on the initial study, it was determined that several prognostic factors influenced the outcomes (Table 12-3). It was also determined that, among selected patients, therapy could be safely discontinued after 4 weeks of amphotericin B 0.3 mg/kg/d and flucytosine 150 mg/kg/d. Selected patients with a good prognosis were patients who were immunocompetent and had no neurologic defects, a lower serum cryptococcal antigen, and an initial white cell count of >20 cells/mm^3 in CSF. Those patients demonstrated an excellent clinical and mycologic response at 4 weeks. After fluconazole became available in the early 1990s, an initial study published by Saag et al in 1992 confirmed the efficacy of fluconazole administered as an initial parenteral dose followed for up to 10 weeks with an oral dose of 200 mg/d. However, although fluconazole was better tolerated than amphotericin B, there was a trend toward more rapid sterilization of CSF in the amphotericin B recipients and no significant difference in overall success. Most importantly, the overall cure rates were disappointing. On the basis of this study, it was concluded that, while fluconazole is an acceptable alternative for initial therapy, it should be reserved for patients who (1) are not critically ill, (2) have a normal mental status at presentation, (3) have no neurologic abnormalities, (4) have a lower fungal burden as determined by a negative CSF India ink study, (5) have a CSF Cryptococcus antigen <1:1,024, and (6) have >20 white cells/mm^3 in CSF. The most important conclusion from the early studies in AIDS patients was that cryptococcal meningitis could be successfully managed with an initial 10-week course of amphotericin B using a minimum dose of 0.3 mg/kg/d, with or without flucytosine, followed by fluconazole at a dose of 200 mg/d.

Based on the findings of this study, a second multicenter study of HIV-infected patients with cryptococcal meningitis was performed. In this study, amphotericin B was used at a higher dose of 0.7 mg/kg/d for the first 2 weeks plus either flucytosine 100 mg/kg/d or placebo (Table 12-4). Although there was no significant difference in the success rates for combination therapy vs monotherapy (60% and 51%, respectively) in the first 2 weeks, there was again a trend toward more rapid mycologic improvement and better overall clinical outcome in the combination therapy arm. Following the initial 2 weeks of therapy, patients were randomized to receive either fluconazole or itraconazole (Sporanox®) for 8 weeks. A similar success rate was seen with both of these regimens (68% and 70%, respectively). However, after patients completed 10 weeks of therapy in the chronic maintenance phase, fluconazole 200 mg/d demonstrated superior efficacy in preventing relapsing cryptococcosis compared with itraconazole 200 mg/d. In addition, patients who initially received amphotericin B plus flucytosine showed lower relapse rates, possibly as a consequence of the penetration of flucytosine into a relatively inaccessible site in the CNS.

There have been relatively few studies in non-HIV-infected individuals. Current recommendations for the treatment of cryptococcal meningitis in HIV-positive patients consist of amphotericin B with flucytosine for 2 weeks, followed by fluconazole 400 mg/d for 6 weeks. This has been proven to result in an 80% response rate in HIV-positive patients and is now recommended for HIV-negative patients.

There have been two small studies in non-HIV-infected patients. One was a prospective study comparing amphotericin B plus flucytosine with an oral regimen consisting of fluconazole 800 mg/d plus flucytosine 100 mg/kg/d for 6 weeks. The study was terminated because of slow patient accrual, but it was apparent that the response to amphotericin B was superior and that the use of amphotericin B in the initial management of this disease is crucial, especially in gravely ill individuals. Use of an oral regimen has a role in mildly ill patients only. In a large retrospective study, Pappas et al reached a similar conclusion endorsing the importance of retaining an amphotericin B-containing regimen as initial treatment, with fluconazole limited to therapy following a significant clinical and mycologic response. Although in vitro amphotericin B susceptibility predicts in vivo response, it is not yet the standard of practice to obtain cryptococcal MICs to antifungals, except in patients with recurrent meningitis where reduced fluconazole (not amphotericin B) has increasingly been reported.

The lipid formulations of amphotericin B have also been used in the treatment of cryptococcal meningitis in

HIV-infected patients. In a large prospective study, liposomal amphotericin B administered at a dose of 3 mg/d, followed by maintenance fluconazole, was shown to be as effective as conventional amphotericin B without the infusion and nephrotoxicity. Posaconazole (Noxafil®) has also shown clinical efficacy in cryptococcal meningitis. Salvage therapy with posaconazole 800 mg/d in divided doses resulted in a successful outcome in 23 of 39 HIV-infected patients.

Because the recurrence rate can be as high as 50%, patients with AIDS who have been successfully treated for an episode of acute cryptococcal meningitis previously had been recommended to take lifelong secondary prophylaxis, which would consist of oral fluconazole 100 to 200 mg daily. However, because immune restoration has now been demonstrated among HIV-infected patients who respond to potent antiretroviral therapy, the risks of reactivation of suppression of opportunistic pathogens has been reassessed. In more recent studies, considerable information has determined that maintenance therapy against *C neoformans* in patients with HIV infection can be interrupted after sustained CD4 counts increase to $>100 \times 10^6$ cells/L for at least 6 months after the start of potent antiretroviral therapy. Nevertheless, patients should be carefully monitored for a sudden decrease in the CD4 count in order to reintroduce suppressive prophylactic regimens. Anticryptococcal therapy should be started in patients whose serum cryptococcal antigen test results revert to positive after discontinuation of maintenance therapy.

Because of its cost, potential drug interactions, and failure to demonstrate survival benefit, primary prophylaxis with fluconazole against *C neoformans* infection in patients with AIDS is not advocated. It is generally recommended that HIV-infected individuals avoid exposure to areas with heavy contamination by avian feces. Adjunctive therapy with interferon-γ along with conventional treatment is being tested in clinical trials. Some benefit has

Table 12-5: Management of Increased Intracranial Pressure

- Management will depend on intracranial OP
  - If OP <180 mm H_2O, observe
  - If OP >180 + symptoms of ↑ ICP, initiate treatment
  - If OP >350 mm H_2O, initiate treatment
- Stepwise management includes:
  - Daily removal of 25-50 cc CSF
  - Temporary lumbar drain
  - Ventriculoperitoneal and lumboperitoneal shunts

CSF= cerebrospinal fluid, ICP = intracranial pressure, OP = opening pressure

emerged in animal models. Similarly, anticryptococcal monoclonal antibodies have been shown to clear cryptococcal polysaccharide antigen from CSF in animal models and are about to be studied in humans.

Management of Raised Intracranial Pressure

Elevated intracranial pressure (Table 12-5) in patients with cryptococcal meningitis is a significant cause of morbidity and mortality. Some of the symptoms and neurologic signs of elevated intracranial pressure can be ameliorated by the removal of CSF via the placement of a lumbar drain. Before a lumbar drain is considered, daily removal of CSF should be performed at the time of a daily spinal tap. At this time, 25 to 50 mL of CSF should be removed to decrease the CSF pressure by approximately 50%. Aggressive use of lumbar puncture reduces the risk of early mortality and late morbidity, especially for patients with extremely high ICP. Multiple LPs and large-volume CSF drainage in HIV-infected patients with elevated ICP are safe after the presence of space-occupying lesions is excluded.

Failure to control the pressure by this means should result in consideration of placement of a lumbar drain. If, after 72 hours of lumbar drainage, the raised intracranial pressure persists, a CSF shunt from the lumbar or ventricular space into the peritoneal cavity should be considered. This approach is indicated for patients whose CNS symptoms have not resolved or who have had transient improvement with symptom recurrence between serial lumbar punctures. Prolonged external lumbar drainage puts patients at risk for bacterial meningitis. The major risk of lumbar drainage results from the presence of a rare coexisting mass lesion and obstructive hydrocephalus, which is a rare complication of cryptococcal meningitis.

Ventriculoperitoneal shunts have shown to be highly effective and safe in HIV-negative patients in Southeast Asia. Occasionally, intraventricular amphotericin B can be delivered through an Ommaya reservoir placed subcutaneously in the scalp, with a catheter located in one of the lateral ventricles. Intraventricular amphotericin B should be reserved for refractory cases in which systemic amphotericin B and other alternatives have failed.

Immune Reconstitution Syndrome

Approximately 10% to 30% of HIV-infected patients coinfected with *Cryptococcus neoformans* who initiate highly active antiretroviral therapy develop immune reconstitution inflammatory syndrome (IRIS). Similarly, 5% of solid organ transplant recipients with *C neoformans* infection develop IRS. The syndrome follows a reduction in or cessation of immunosuppressive therapy, corresponding to a reversal of a predominantly Th2 response at the onset of infection to a Th1 pro-inflammatory response. The clinical syndromes include culture-negative meningitis, inflammatory lymphadenitis, necrotizing pneumonitis, and cryptococcomas. Differentiating IRS meningitis from relapsed *C neoformans* meningitis in patients treated with HAART can be difficult. In addition to negative CSF cultures, the *Cryptococcus*-related type is associated with higher CSF opening pressures, higher glucose IRS levels, and higher WBC counts compared with typical HIV-associated *C neoformans* meningitis. An essential component of diagnosis is a recent start in ART with concurrent reduction in plasma viremia of greater than 1 log, and increased CD4 counts. Management with corticosteroids (1 mg/kg/d) and antifungals is recommended although controlled studies are lacking.

Suggested Readings

Buchanan KL, Murphy JW: What makes *Cryptococcus neoformans* a pathogen? *Emerg Infect Dis* 1998;4:71-83.

Hamill RJ: Cryptococcal meningitis. *Curr Treat Options Infect Dis* 2001;3:129-136.

Liliang PC, Liang CL, Chang WN, et al: Use of ventriculoperitoneal shunts to treat uncontrollable intracranial hypertension in patients who have cryptococcal meningitis without hydrocephalus. *Clin Infect Dis* 2002;34:E64-E68.

Mussini C, Pezzotti P, Miro JM, et al: Discontinuation of maintenance therapy for cryptococcal meningitis in patients with AIDS treated with highly active antiretroviral therapy: an international observational study. *Clin Infect Dis* 2004;38:565-571.

Pappas PG: Therapy of cryptococcal meningitis in non-HIV-infected patients. *Curr Infect Dis Rep* 2001;3:365-370.

Rozenbaum R, Goncalves AJ: Clinical epidemiological study of 171 cases of cryptococcosis. *Clin Infect Dis* 1994;18:369-380.

Saag MS, Graybill RJ, Larsen RA, et al: Practice guidelines for the management of cryptococcal disease. Infectious Diseases Society of America. *Clin Infect Dis* 2000;30:710-718.

Shelburne SA 3rd, Darcourt J, White AC Jr, et al: The role of immune reconstitution inflammatory syndrome in AIDS-related

Cryptococcus neoformans disease in the era of highly active antiretroviral therapy. *Clin Infect Dis* 2005;40:1049-1052.

Sorrell TC: Cryptococcus neoformans variety gattii. *Med Mycol* 2001;39:155-168.

Chapter 13

Aspergillosis

Aspergillus species are found worldwide and are ubiquitous in the environment. Aspergillosis encompasses a broad spectrum of diseases caused by members of the genus *Aspergillus*. The clinical manifestation and severity of the disease depend upon the immunologic state of the patient.

In the last decade, there have been significant advances in the diagnosis and treatment of invasive aspergillosis. However, invasive aspergillosis remains a major cause of morbidity and mortality in immunosuppressed patients. Lowered host resistance due to such factors as underlying debilitating disease, neutropenia, chemotherapy, immunosuppressive agents, antimicrobial agents, and steroids predisposes the patients to colonization, invasive disease, or both. Additionally, aspergillosis is occasionally seen as an opportunistic pathogen in patients with bronchiectasis, carcinoma, sarcoidosis, or tuberculosis.

Epidemiology

Aspergillus species are ubiquitous saprophytes found worldwide in nature. *Aspergillus* species are one of the most common organisms found in compost piles and readily isolated from the soil, air, water, and food. It is frequently isolated from hospital ventilation systems and hospital construction sites. In addition, it may also be found in 1% to 16% of respiratory secretions in a normal host. There are approximately 600 recognized species of *Aspergillus*,

Table 13-1: Distribution of *Aspergillus* Species

***Aspergillus* species**	**Isolation Frequency (%)**
A fumigatus	66
A flavus	14
A niger	7
A terreus	4
A versicolor	2
A nidulans	1
A oryzae	1
A glaucus	1
A ustus	<1

of which *A fumigatus* is the most frequent cause of disease in humans, followed by *A flavus*, *A niger* and, occasionally, *A terreus*, *A nidulans*, and *A glaucus* (Table 13-1). Aspergilli are molds that reproduce by means of spores termed conidia. Hyphae are septate and dichotomously branched. If the infection rapidly progresses, the hyphae tend to be of even diameter; in indolent infections, the hyphae have bullous, widened areas. Sporulation is rarely observed, but aspergilli grow well in stored hay or grain, decayed vegetation, and soil. Invasive infection is rare unless a marked immunodeficiency is present.

Aspergillus is the second most common cause of fungal disease in hematopoietic stem cell transplant (HSCT) recipients, solid organ transplant recipients, and hematologic and other cancers. In general, infection occurs in severely immunocompromised hosts, particularly in HSCT patients who develop graft-vs-host disease (GVHD), patients who develop prolonged and profound neutropenia, or patients with neutrophil dysfunction from corticosteroid therapy

Table 13-2: Predisposing Factors for Aspergillosis

Major Risk Factors	*Minor Risk Factors*
• Neutropenia • Graft-vs-host disease (GVHD) • Cytomegalovirus infection/reactivation • Hematopoietic stem cell transplants • Solid organ transplants – Lung transplant – Heart transplant – Liver transplants • Steroids >1 mg/kg/d systemic or inhaled • Hematologic malignancies	• COPD on steroids • Cirrhosis • Burns • Solid organ malignancies • Immunosuppressants – Cyclosporine – Methotrexate – Azathioprine – Cyclophosphamide • IVDU • Advanced HIV CD4 cell counts <50 mm^3 • IV drug use • Occasionally may coexist with gram-negative bacterial pneumonias

(Table 13-2). Outbreaks in hospitals from renovations, new constructions, and ventilation systems have been reported frequently.

Similarly, patients with chronic granulomatous disease (CGD) may present with invasive aspergillosis because of the inability of their phagocytes to generate microbicidal substrates. Less frequently, patients with alcoholic cirrhosis, collagen vascular diseases, and post-influenza infection are also at risk to develop invasive aspergillosis, and even nonimmunocompromised hosts may infrequently develop disseminated aspergillosis.

Pathogenesis

Aspergillus is acquired by inhalation of airborne spores; these spores (conidia) are small enough to reach alveoli or sinuses. Occasionally, conidia in operating rooms may enter the implantation site of prosthetic valves. Exposure is universal, but disease is uncommon because host factors are very important. Keeping the immunocompromised host away from dusty hospital renovation or construction areas is useful, as is keeping potted plants out of patient hospital rooms. *Aspergillus* species, like many other molds, are considered angioinvasive pathogens. In other words, they have a tendency for vascular invasion, producing thrombosis, ischemia, infarction, and tissue necrosis. In a compromised host, vascular invasion is paramount, leading to infarction, necrosis, edema, and hemorrhage in distal tissues. Hyphae are abundant in infected tissues, even forming radially branching clusters. In contrast, vascular invasion is not seen, and hyphae are sparse in tissue from patients with CGD.

Host defenses rely on phagocytes, not upon antibodies or lymphocytes. Complement facilitates neutrophil damage to hyphae and monocyte killing of conidia. In addition, oxidation killing is important because CGD patients have increased risk of infection.

Most infections originate in the respiratory tract, then subsequently disseminate via the bloodstream to other tissues, including other respiratory tract sites, the central nervous system (CNS), kidneys, eyes, skin, liver, and spleen. Accordingly, the respiratory tract is the most commonly involved site (56%), followed by the CNS (6%), and the upper respiratory tract (sinuses) and skin (5%). Multiorgan involvement or disseminated infection is found in about 20% of patients.

Table 13-3: Mortality Rates in Aspergillosis

Underlying Disease/Condition	Mortality Rate (%)
CNS or disseminated infection	88
Bone marrow transplantation	86
Respiratory tract	59
Leukemia/lymphoma	49
Overall mortality	*58*

Prognosis depends on the type and severity of disease and the underlying immunologic status of the patient. Invasion from a cutaneous source, such as central venous catheters, rarely occurs.

The outcome of infection also depends on the site of infection and the status of the underlying immunosuppressive disease (Table 13-3).

Clinical Manifestations

Aspergillus infection can manifest in a variety of ways, ranging from colonization to life-threatening invasive disease (Table 13-4). Moreover, the clinical manifestations depend on the route of infection and the underlying disease. The overall mortality rate depends on the underlying immunosuppressive state, and can vary from 40% to 90%.

Ear

Otomycosis is caused by the growth of mold in the external ear canal, which is common, but rarely invasive. Generally, the fungus grows as a saprophyte in debris and cerumen. Treatment is directed at the underlying cause, which is frequently chronic otitis externa and not the *Aspergillus*.

Table 13-4: Manifestations of Invasive Aspergillosis

- Fever
- Pulmonary symptomatology
  - pleuritic chest pain–pleural rub
  - dry cough
  - dyspnea
  - hemoptysis—usually minor, occasionally catastrophic
- Chest x-ray—early may be normal, later followed by infiltrates-infarction, nodules-cavitation
- Focal neurologic lesions
  - seizures
  - focal neurologic deficits
- Systemic, multiorgan dysfunction
- Hemorrhagic skin lesions
- Negative blood cultures (~99%)

Paranasal Sinuses (Sinusitis)

Acute paranasal sinusitis occurs primarily in patients with neutropenia (Figure 13-1; see color plate insert). Sinusitis is initially indistinguishable from bacterial sinusitis and may actually coexist. In neutropenic patients, mucosal invasion begins in the nasal mucosa or sinuses and may spread rapidly to contiguous structures, causing vascular invasion and necrosis. It rarely affects a competent host, and when it does, the disease is indolent, granulomatous, and uncommonly becomes invasive.

Manifestations include headaches, sinus pain rapidly complicated by proptosis, and monocular blindness. Fungal sinusitis also occurs in patients with a history of allergic rhinitis, chronic nasal congestion, or recurrent sinusitis.

Aspergillus or other molds may be found in the sinus mucosal secretions, along with eosinophils, granulocytes, and Charcot-Leyden crystals in a noninvasive form.

In allergic fungal sinusitis, the natural course is poorly defined, and on occasion may form a fungus ball in the sinus cavities.

Diagnosis is established by the identification of hyphae in tissue. However, in the high-risk patient, a presumptive diagnosis can be established by the identification of *Aspergillus* species from nasal or sinus cultures.

Endophthalmitis

Ocular infection or endophthalmitis is generally produced by direct inoculation after either surgery or trauma, and may be followed by deep stromal invasion. Occasionally, endophthalmitis may be of hematogenous origin, as is seen in neutropenics or intravenous (IV) drug users with endocarditis.

Allergic Bronchopulmonary Aspergillosis (ABPA)

Allergic bronchopulmonary aspergillosis is a chronic disease progressing from episodes of acute corticosteroid-responsive asthma to fibrotic end-stage lung disease. This is thought to be due to a hypersensitivity reaction to *Aspergillus* in the bronchial tree without tissue invasion.

Most patients have a history of pre-existing asthma with fleeting pulmonary infiltrates caused by bronchial plugging. A set of defined criteria have been developed to assist in making the diagnosis: (1) episodic bronchial obstruction (asthma); (2) eosinophilia; (3) positive immediate (type 1) skin test to *Aspergillus* antigen; (4) elevated total IgE and IgG antibodies specific to *A fumigatus*; (5) elevated serum IgE concentrations; (6) precipitating serum antibodies against *Aspergillus* antigens; (7) history of pulmonary infiltrates; and (8) episodic bronchial plugging that leads to central areas of saccular bronchiectasis. Patients occasionally have a history of expectorating brown mucous plugs that are microscopically positive for hyphae. Sputum cultures may be positive for *Aspergillus* in about two thirds of patients. Some patients experience no permanent damage, while others may develop steroid-dependent asthma or irreversible COPD.

Chest x-rays frequently reveal alveolar infiltrates, perihilar densities, atelectasis, and cavitary lesions. Infiltrates tend to be transient with a predilection for the upper lobes.

Aspergillomas (Fungus Balls)

Aspergillomas consist of hyphal elements, fibrin, mucus, amorphous debris, host's tissues, and a few inflammatory cells. They are generally seen in patients with pre-existing cavities or underlying lung disease such as tuberculosis (TB), cancer, sarcoidosis, histoplasmosis, bullous emphysema, or bronchiectasis.

Clinically, 75% of patients present with hemoptysis, and it disappears spontaneously in approximately 10% of patients. The diagnosis is suspected in a high-risk patient with positive sputum cultures on chest x-ray. Aspergillomas tend to be solitary, average 3 to 5 cm, and consist of an intracavitary mass partially surrounded by a radiolucent crescent with walls of varying thickness.

Sputum smears and cultures are only intermittently positive for *Aspergillus*, found in approximately 50% of patients. Serum *Aspergillus* precipitins are positive in about 90% of cases.

Complications include spread to pleura, broncho-pleural fistulas, bacterial lung abscess, superinfections, and rarely, osteomyelitis that primarily affects the thoracic vertebrae.

Invasive Pulmonary Aspergillosis

Invasive pulmonary involvement by *Aspergillus* species is characterized by fever, nonproductive cough or hemoptysis, tachypnea, and variable pulmonary infiltrates on x-ray, which may be unimpressive during neutropenia.

Molds, such as *Aspergillus* species, frequently invade blood vessels, inducing pulmonary infarcts accompanied by chest pain, pleuritic rubs, and segmental pulmonary infiltrates. Chest x-rays may reveal single or multiple lesions that may be nodular or cavitary. A computed tomography (CT) scan of the chest is more sensitive than chest x-ray in detecting early infection, and often reveals multiple ring-enhancing cavitary lesions that accompany relatively unimpressive nondiagnostic chest x-rays. A suggestive diagnosis may be made on the basis of a halo surrounding a denser consolidated area or an air-crescent sign.

In immunocompromised hosts, pulmonary aspergillosis can extend to involve the pericardium or disseminate hematogenously to cause endocarditis and CNS disease presenting as focal neurologic disease, including seizures.

A subacute or chronic form of invasive pulmonary aspergillosis presents as a slowly progressive necrotizing pulmonary lesion characterized by persistent antibiotic-resistant fever, hemoptysis, and debilitation. This form of aspergillosis has been most often seen in patients with AIDS, diabetes, and CGD.

Invasive Aspergillosis

The incidence of invasive aspergillosis has increased greatly during the past 15 years. The increase is multifactorial and due to new and more potent immunosuppressive regimens, greater number of immunocompromised patients, use of potent broad-spectrum antimicrobials, use of high-dose corticosteroids, and the increase in bone marrow and solid organ transplant recipients.

If bone marrow function does not return, widespread dissemination to other organs can occur, primarily to other parts of lung, brain, liver, spleen, heart, and thyroid. Invasive aspergillosis must be strongly considered in the high-risk patient with neutropenia, fever, and pulmonary infiltrates that fail to respond to broad-spectrum antibacterial therapy. A frequent triad includes a HSCT patient who develops GVHD, is taking high-dose steroids (prednisone 1 mg/kg/d), and develops CMV antigenemia.

The manifestations of aspergillosis in CGD patients are different from those found in neutropenic patients. The symptoms are insidious and include fever, pulmonary infiltrates, increased erythrocyte sedimentation rate, a chest x-ray with an area of pneumonia, or many small nodular infiltrates. Spread to the thoracic spine, pleura, ribs, brain, and skin is not uncommon.

Aspergillosis of the Central Nervous System

The CNS is one of the most common sites of infection, which has been estimated to occur here between 10% to 20% of the time in invasive aspergillosis. Compromised hosts may have cerebral vessels occluded by *Aspergillus*, causing cerebral infarction with necrosis and occasionally hemorrhages. A brain abscess is the most common presentation. There are four primary types of CNS aspergillosis: meningitis, meningoencephalitis, and single or multiple brain abscesses. Clinical symptoms include rapidly developing stroke syndrome, seizures, altered mentation, and progressive obtundation. Surgical intervention frequently finds an area of necrosis with numerous hyphae surrounded by dense granulation tissue. Despite the newer antifungals, the mortality rate of CNS infection is still high, > 80%. Recently, however, using the new azole, voriconazole (Vfend®), several investigators have been able to demonstrate response rates of about 25%.

Endocarditis

Aspergilli may infect normal, damaged, or prosthetic valves. *Aspergillus* species may infect heart valves during surgery, or rarely, during hematogenous dissemination in intravenous drug users. Patients present with fever, cerebral emboli, heart failure, or conduction defects. Despite the endovascular focus of infection, the fungus is rarely cultured from blood. The manifestations are similar to those seen with bacterial endocarditis, and the diagnosis is frequently made post mortem.

Gastrointestinal Tract

The stomach, esophagus, small intestine, and colon are frequent sites of infection. The lesions are caused either by direct invasion from the mucosal lining or hematogenous spread from invasive disease. The necrotic lesions tend to extend from the mucosa into the muscularis and produce gastrointestinal ulcerations, primarily in compromised hosts. Subsequently, vascular invasion with resultant thrombosis and infarction may result in gastrointestinal bleeds.

Cutaneous Aspergillosis

Cutaneous infections are primarily seen in neutropenic, severely immunocompromised hosts, and are frequently a marker of disseminated disease. Occasionally, they may also be seen in burns, IV sites, and surgical wounds. The resulting infection may be caused by direct inoculation of *Aspergillus* from an environmental source or occur secondary to hematogenous dissemination. The lesion is classically a necrotizing skin ulceration, covered with a black eschar (Figure 13-2; see color plate insert). For unknown reasons, the lesions tend to be seen more commonly in the lower extremities.

Aspergillus Osteomyelitis

Aspergillus bone infection is uncommon but is usually seen in neutropenic patients, IV drug users, or CGD patients. The infection begins by contiguous spread to rib or vertebrae, or by hematogenous spread to vertebrae in compromised hosts. Occasionally, disk space infection with an associated epidural abscess occurs.

Diagnosis

The diagnosis of invasive aspergillosis continues to be a significant problem. In fact, the diagnosis is frequently

Table 13-5: Problems With Diagnosis of Aspergillosis

- Nonspecific signs and symptoms
- Nonspecific laboratory parameters
- Difficulty establishing colonization vs invasion
- Blood cultures rarely positive (<1%)
- Need to establish tissue invasion and need for biopsy
- *Aspergillus* species grow slowly in vitro
- Nonculture detection test not reliable

made using clinical manifestations and histopathologic analysis of affected tissue. Early recognition of the hosts at greatest risk (prolonged neutropenia, GVHD, corticosteroid usage, CMV antigenemia, etc) is the key to early diagnosis and subsequent therapy (Table 13-5). Definitive diagnosis of aspergillosis is very difficult because there are no pathognomonic laboratory findings other than cultures of biopsy material from infected tissue and histopathology. The gold standard in establishing a diagnosis of invasive aspergillosis is the demonstration of tissue invasion from hyphae and a positive culture for *Aspergillus*.

The early initiation of appropriate antifungal therapy is crucial in the management of this infection. Thus, efforts have focused on noninvasive studies to establish a putative diagnosis of invasive aspergillosis. In a high-risk patient, especially with prolonged neutropenia, GVHD, high-dose steroids, and a positive culture from the nares, sputum, or bronchoalveolar lavage are predictive of invasive disease and strong enough evidence to initiate early presumptive antifungal therapy (Table 13-6). In the low-risk patient with CGD, HIV infection or steroid use, tissue biopsy of an infected site is strongly encouraged

Table 13-6: Criteria for Empiric Antifungal Therapy for Presumptive Invasive Aspergillosis

High-Risk Patients—
Start Empirical Treatment if:

- Neutropenia
- *Aspergillus* species isolated
- Fever
- Lung infiltrates or compatible computed tomography findings

Low-Risk Patients—
Biopsy and then Start Therapy if:

- Solid organ transplantation
- Cancer
- Chronic granulomatous disease
- HIV positive

before initiating antifungal therapy. The development of diagnostic criteria has been very difficult. Recently, however, criteria for patients with hematologic cancer, other cancer, and bone marrow transplantation have been developed.

Although the isolation of *Aspergillus* from tissue is the gold standard, and because fungal smears and cultures are frequently negative, noninvasive indirect evidence of invasive aspergillosis has been evaluated by serology. There are two testing methods available. The galactomannan enzyme-linked immunosorbent assay (ELISA) assay has been used in Europe for several years and uses a monoclonal antibody to galactomannan antigen. Galactomannan is a constituent of the *Aspergillus* cell wall found in the serum of patients with invasive disease. The current ELISA lowers the detection limit range to 0.5-1.0 ng/mL of galactomannan in the serum. According to Maertens et al, the reported sensitivity is approximately 90%, with a specificity of 81% to 100%, and a positive predictive value of 80%. Serial monitoring increases the sensitivity of the assay, and may detect disease before clinical suspicion. False positives can occur up to 10 days after the start of antifungal therapy and also in association with the use of certain antimicrobials such as piperacillin/tazobactam (Zosyn®IV). Furthermore, a recent study has demonstrated a decrease in the sensitivity of the galactomannan assay if the patient has been receiving either prophylactic or empiric antifungal therapy. In addition, it is also possible to use the assay as a therapeutic monitoring test of antifungal efficacy.

The second nonculture detection assay is the Fungitell Assay, an amebocyte lysis assay that detects 1,3 β-D glucan, a product of fungal cell walls of several fungal organisms, in the serum. It has been available in the US since 2004. In prospective clinical trials, the assay has a sensitivity of 70% to 80%, with a specificity of 80% to 98%. It is, however, considered a panfungal assay, because it is able to detect a broad spectrum of fungi, including *Fusarium, Trichosporon, Saccharomyces, Acremonium*, in addition to *Aspergillus* and *Candida* species.

Plain radiographs are frequently used to establish the diagnosis. However, plain radiographs are often insensitive and miss subtle pulmonary findings. A high-definition CT scan of the thorax may be very beneficial in establishing the diagnosis of invasive pulmonary aspergillosis in the patient with a HSCT. This includes patients with completely normal chest x-rays. The high definition or spiral CT of the thorax may identify small nodules, cavities, or infiltrates prior to the chest x-ray developing any abnormalities. The infiltrates are frequently nodular and peripherally located. During early infection, the nodule is surrounded by a "halo," an area of intermediate attenuation. After approximately 1 week, the halo disappears and the infiltrate becomes less defined, followed by the appearance of the "crescent" sign when cavitation takes place.

Bronchoscopy with bronchoalveolar lavage and a transbronchial biopsy may be able to detect about 50% of histologically proven cases of aspergillosis. However, the use of invasive procedures in patients who are thrombocytopenic often cannot be performed.

Histology of infected tissue demonstrates angular (45°), dichotomously branching septate hyphae, which are characteristic for *Aspergillus* species. However, this may also be compatible with infection from other molds such as *Fusarium, Scedosporium*, and *Zygomycetes*.

Recently, molecular diagnostic assays, specifically polymerase chain reaction (PCR), DNA fingerprinting, and DNA probes have been used in an attempt to use noninvasive testing for the diagnosis of invasive aspergillosis. Their usefulness is based on the assays being sensitive and specific, rapid, reproducible, and capable of detecting small amounts of fungal DNA, even though growth may be delayed 1 to 2 weeks or does not occur at all. Unfortunately, these assays are still in the early stages of development.

Treatment

The management and prognosis of aspergillosis depend on the specific form of disease and the degree of immune suppression (Table 13-7 and Table 13-8). For more than 45 years, amphotericin B deoxycholate (Fungizone®) was the mainstay of antifungal therapy for aspergillosis. Recent studies by Herbrecht et al have demonstrated that therapy with voriconazole leads to improved survival when compared to amphotericin B in invasive aspergillosis, without the dose-limiting nephrotoxicity that is so commonly seen with amphotericin B. Furthermore, guidelines for the management of aspergillosis have been published by the Infectious Diseases Society of America.

Table 13-7: Treatment of Aspergillosis

Agent	Initial Dose
Voriconazole (Vfend®)	6 mg/kg IV q 12 h x 2 doses, followed by 4 mg/kg IV q 12 h
	400 mg PO q 12 h x 2 doses, followed by 300 mg PO q 12 h
Caspofungin (Cancidas®)	70 mg IV x 1 dose, followed by 50 mg IV q.d.
Amphotericin B deoxycholate (Amphocin®, Fungizone®)	0.8-1.25 mg/kg/d IV
Itraconazole (Sporanox®)	200 mg t.i.d. for 4 d, then 200 mg b.i.d. PO
Liposomal amphotericin B (AmBisome®)	5 mg/kg/d IV
Amphotericin B lipid complex (Abelcet®)	5 mg/kg/d IV

Newer pharmacokinetic studies demonstrate significant patient-to-patient differences among the different azole antifungals. A significant amount of literature recommends therapeutic drug monitoring of the azoles, especially itraconazole, voriconazole, and posaconazole.

Allergic Bronchopulmonary Aspergillosis

The goal of therapy for allergic bronchopulmonary aspergillosis (ABPA) should include relief of bronchospasm, reversal of the parenchymal infiltration, and preservation

Comments

Considered first-line therapy; visual events described in 20% to 30% of patients

Approved for patients with refractory disease

Considered first-line therapy but high failure rate; significant interaction with cyclosporine

Useful if a patient is eating and not receiving cytochrome P-450 inducers; significant interaction with cyclosporine; levels should be measured to ensure adequate absorption

Less nephrotoxic than amphotericin B deoxycholate

Less nephrotoxic than amphotericin B deoxycholate

of lung structure and function. Corticosteroids have been the mainstay of therapy for many years but steroid use has many pitfalls. The recommended dosage is 0.5 mg/kg/d during exacerbations until the chest x-ray clears, and for at least 3 months. Once the patient is stable, the steroid dose should be tapered over 3 months, if possible. A study conducted by the Mycoses Study Group demonstrated that itraconazole (Sporanox®) 200 mg b.i.d. has been successfully used to decrease airflow obstruction episodes and decrease exacerbations without the use of steroid therapy.

Table 13-8: Treatment Options for Aspergillosis Infections

Infection	Primary Therapy
Invasive pulmonary aspergillosis and tracheobronchial aspergillosis	Voriconazole 6 mg/kg IV q 12 h, followed by 4 mg/kg; oral dose is 200 mg b.i.d.
Chronic necrotizing aspergillosis (subacute invasive pulmonary aspergillosis)	Voriconazole 6 mg/kg IV q 12 h, followed by 4 mg/kg; oral dose is 200 mg b.i.d.
CNS aspergillosis	Voriconazole 6 mg/kg IV q 12 h, followed by 4 mg/kg; oral dose is 200 mg b.i.d.
Invasive aspergillus sinusitis	Voriconazole 6 mg/kg IV q 12 h, followed by 4 mg/kg; oral dose is 200 mg b.i.d.

Secondary Therapy	Salvage Therapy
Liposomal amphotericin B 5 mg/kg/d	Amphotericin B lipid complex injection 5 mg/kg/d; itraconazole 2.5 mg/kg of oral solution b.i.d.; caspofungin 70 mg loading dose, followed by 50 mg/d; posaconazole oral solution 400 mg b.i.d.
Liposomal amphotericin B 5 mg/kg/d; itraconazole 2.5 mg/kg of oral solution b.i.d.	Amphotericin B lipid complex injection 5 mg/kg/d; caspofungin 70 mg loading dose, followed by 50 mg/d; posaconazole oral solution 400 mg b.i.d.
Liposomal amphotericin B 5 mg/kg/d	Amphotericin B lipid complex injection 5 mg/kg/d; itraconazole 2.5 mg/kg of oral solution b.i.d.; caspofungin 70 mg loading dose, followed by 50 mg/d; posaconazole oral solution 400 mg b.i.d.
Liposomal amphotericin B 5 mg/kg/d; itraconazole 2.5 mg/kg of oral solution b.i.d.	Amphotericin B lipid complex injection 5 mg/kg/d; caspofungin 70 mg loading dose, followed by 50 mg/d; posaconazole oral solution 400 mg b.i.d.

Table 13-8: Treatment Options for Aspergillosis Infections *(continued)*

Infection	Primary Therapy
Osteoarticular aspergillosis	Voriconazole 6 mg/kg IV q 12 h, followed by 4 mg/kg; oral dose is 200 mg b.i.d.
Cardiac aspergillosis	Voriconazole 6 mg/kg IV q 12 h, followed by 4 mg/kg; oral dose is 200 mg b.i.d.
Aspergilloma	None, occasionally may need surgical resection
Allergic broncho-pulmonary aspergillosis	Itraconazole 200 mg b.i.d.
Allergic aspergillus sinusitis	Itraconazole 200 mg PO b.i.d.

Secondary Therapy	Salvage Therapy
Liposomal amphotericin B 5 mg/kg/d; itraconazole 2.5 mg/kg of oral solution b.i.d.	Amphotericin B lipid complex injection 5 mg/kg/d; caspofungin 70 mg loading dose, followed by 50 mg/d; posaconazole oral solution 400 mg b.i.d.
Liposomal amphotericin B 5 mg/kg/d; itraconazole 2.5 mg/kg of oral solution b.i.d.	Amphotericin B lipid complex injection 5 mg/kg/d; caspofungin 70 mg loading dose, followed by 50 mg/d; posaconazole oral solution 400 mg b.i.d.
Voriconazole 6 mg/kg IV q 12 h, followed by 4 mg/kg; oral dose is 200 mg b.i.d.	
Voriconazole 6 mg/kg IV q 12 h, followed by 4 mg/kg; oral dose is 200 mg b.i.d.; or posaconazole 400 mg PO b.i.d.	

(continued on next page)

Aspergilloma

In most situations, patients do not require any form of therapy. Aspergillomas may be treated by surgical resection. However, this approach may cause significant morbidity and mortality and therefore should be reserved for patients who develop severe hemoptysis. Systemic antifungal therapy is rarely curative because of poor penetration of drug into the fungus ball.

Invasive Aspergillosis

The management of invasive aspergillosis has changed markedly over the last 5 years. However, despite newer antifungal therapy, the mortality rates still range from 50% to 100%, depending primarily on the underlying disease and the site of infection.

The current mainstay of therapy for invasive aspergillosis is now considered to be voriconazole (Vfend®). The appropriate dose of voriconazole for aspergillosis is 6 mg/kg b.i.d. for 1 day, followed by 4 mg/kg b.i.d. A recently published, randomized, multicenter study compared conventional amphotericin B and voriconazole as initial therapy for invasive aspergillosis. This pivotal study in patients with invasive aspergillosis demonstrated that initial therapy with voriconazole led to better responses and improved survival with fewer serious side effects, specifically renal insufficiency and infusion-related toxicity.

Voriconazole is one of the newer lipophilic triazole antifungals, structurally related to fluconazole. It exhibits excellent in vitro activity against a broad range of fungi, including *Candida albicans*, non-*albicans Candida* species, *Aspergillus, Fusarium,* and *Scedosporium apiospermum*. Its oral bioavailability is >95%, thus, it may be used orally. Less than 2% of the drug is excreted unchanged in the urine. Adverse events include skin rashes in 10% to 18% of patients, elevations in aspartate transaminase (AST), alanine transaminase (ALT), total bilirubin, and alkaline phosphatase in 4% to 20% of patients and transient visual disturbances that are described in 20% to 30% of patients.

Amphotericin B (deoxycholate or lipid preparations) continues to be the alternative antifungal agent for invasive aspergillosis. Amphotericin B deoxycholate can be administered parenterally at a dosage varying from 1.0 to 1.5 mg/kg/d for a total dose of 1.5 to 4.0 g. Many *Aspergillus* species are relatively insensitive to amphotericin B, so results are poor. In addition, *A terreus* is considered intrinsically resistant to the polyenes. Amphotericin B's adverse events include nephrotoxicity, which occurs in 30% to 40% of patients receiving parenteral amphotericin B. Given the long duration of therapy required in most patients, nephrotoxicity is predictable. Electrolyte abnormalities include the depletion of potassium and magnesium and are seen in almost 100% of patients. Infusion-related toxicity occasionally occurs in the form of acute reactions about 30 to 45 minutes after beginning infusion. If therapy lasts for more than 1 week, it is essential to monitor complete blood count with differential 3 times/wk while the patient is on therapy.

The lipid preparations of amphotericin B, which facilitate the administration of much higher doses with fewer side effects, have also shown encouraging results in studies of refractory aspergillosis. The three amphotericin B lipid preparations (Amphotec®, Abelcet®, AmBisome®) are FDA approved. All appear to deliver higher concentrations of the drug with a theoretical increase in therapeutic potential and decreased nephrotoxicity. Although all are lipid formulations of amphotericin B, the different formulations are not interchangeable and dosages may vary (Table 13-7). Although significantly less than with conventional amphotericin B, the lipid preparations still have important side effects. Nephrotoxicity, although less than with d-amphotericin B, still occurs in 15% to 25% of patients. Infusion-related toxicity also occurs. Elevations in hepatic transaminases, alkaline phosphatases, and serum bilirubin may occasionally occur.

Itraconazole is also approved for use in aspergillosis, but has had limited use. It has shown efficacy in patients with aspergilloma, chronic necrotizing pulmonary aspergillosis, ABPA, and invasive aspergillosis. Itraconazole in vitro exhibits activity against a broad spectrum of fungi, including *Candida albicans* and many non-*albicans Candida* species, and *Aspergillus* species. Both the oral solution and injection contain itraconazole solubilized by hydroxypropyl-β-cyclodextrin as a molecular inclusion complex. The dosage for aspergillosis is 100 to 300 mg PO twice daily. In severe, life-threatening infections, the loading dose is 200 mg t.i.d. for the first 3 days, followed by 200 mg b.i.d. The oral bioavailability is maximized when the drug is taken with food. Itraconazole is extensively distributed into tissues, especially the lungs, brain, kidneys, liver, spleen, bone, and muscle, where the drug concentrations are 2 to 3 times higher than the corresponding plasma concentration. The compound is metabolized by the liver into many metabolites, including hydroxy-itraconazole, the major metabolite, which possesses in vitro activity similar to the parent compound. Renal excretion of parent drug is <1%. Antacids may reduce absorption of itraconazole. Edema may occur with coadministration of calcium channel blockers (eg, amlodipine, and nifedipine). Rhabdomyolysis has been reported with the coadministration of HMG-CoA reductase inhibitors (lovastatin [Mevacor®] or simvastatin [Zocor®]). Nausea, vomiting, diarrhea, and abdominal discomfort are the more common side effects.

Caspofungin (Cancidas®) is the first of the new family of antifungal compounds—a semisynthetic, water-soluble pneumocandin derived from the fermentation products of *Glarea lozoyensis*. These drugs are noncompetitive inhibitors of the synthesis of the enzyme glucan synthase, which produces (1,3)-β-D-glucan, an essential component of the cell wall of susceptible fungi. Caspofungin possesses in vitro activity against a broad range of fungi, including *C albicans*, many non-*albicans Candida* species, and *A fu-*

migatus, A flavus, and *A terreus*. The recommended dose is 70 mg IV loading dose, followed by 50 mg IV daily. Distribution instead of excretion or biotransformation is the primary mechanism influencing plasma clearance. There is minimal renal excretion and some hepatic metabolism by hydrolysis and N-acetylation. Less than 2% of dose is excreted unchanged in the urine. Caspofungin reduces tacrolimus levels by approximately 20%, while cyclosporine increases caspofungin levels by approximately 35%. Co-administration of both have led to transient increases in transaminases in about 10% of patients. The more common side effects include phlebitis/thrombophlebitis (11% to 15%), liver function test abnormalities (AST, ALT, and alkaline phosphatase, 10% to 13%), and infusion-related toxicity (10%). In patients with moderate hepatic insufficiency, after a loading dose of 70 mg, a daily dose of 35 mg should be used. Since there is minimal renal excretion, the daily dosage does not have to be modified for patients in renal failure. Caspofungin was the first echinocandin compound approved for use in the treatment of invasive aspergillosis in patients who are refractory to, or intolerant of, other antifungals.

Several drugs such as posaconazole and micafungin, and a new FDA approved agent, anidulafungin (Eraxis™), have demonstrated in vitro activity against *Aspergillus* species and are being extensively evaluated. In a recent multicenter study of patients with invasive aspergillosis who were refractory to, or intolerant of, conventional therapy, posaconazole therapy was found to have a higher success rate (42% vs 26%; $P = 0.006$), and improved survival compared with the control group.

In the past, combination therapy has been occasionally used in patients with invasive aspergillosis. In an early clinical trial, the combination of high-dose amphotericin B (1.0 to 1.5 mg/kg) together with flucytosine, dosed to achieve a peak serum level of 30 to 60 µg/mL, was associated with a higher survival rate (87%) in patients with leukemia and invasive aspergillosis. Other combinations included the addition of rifampin (Rifadin®, Rifadin®IV) to amphotericin B due to reports demonstrating some degree of in vitro synergistic activity with this combination of drugs. Most of the time however, the adverse events limited their combined use.

The recent approval of new antifungals with different mechanisms of action have increased our interest in the use of combination antifungals. Recent in vitro and animal trials have suggested some in vitro additive or synergistic effect with the combination of echinocandins (caspofungin, anidulafungin, micafungin [Mycamine®]) and either voriconazole or amphotericin B. Controlled clinical trials, however, have not been undertaken. At this point, although frequently used in clinical practice, combination antifungal therapy does not have any definitive research to unequivocally support its standardized use.

Although the role of immunoadjuvants for invasive fungal infections has not been well studied, several anecdotal reports have occasionally demonstrated improved outcomes. Future research using G-CSF, GM-CSF, and interferon to help augment host response to fungal infections may prove beneficial in managing these opportunistic pathogens and improving outcome.

Surgical therapy, either alone or in combination with antifungal chemotherapy, may also be useful in selected patients with either localized pulmonary or CNS aspergillosis. Surgical excision may be useful in brain abscess and sinus infections from *Aspergillus*. In addition, valve replacement is mandatory in managing *Aspergillus* endocarditis. For patients with aspergilloma, surgery may be required if massive hemoptysis develops; otherwise, patients may continue to be followed with close observation. Indications for surgery include diagnostic resection, disease reduction, and massive hemoptysis from a single lesion. Surgical resection, however, does have risks such as hemorrhage.

A crucial factor in optimizing therapy in any patient with invasive aspergillosis is the decrease or elimination of the immunosuppression whenever possible.

The recent literature suggests that if patients are diagnosed and treated early with appropriate antifungal therapy, the response rates may reach 50% or greater.

Prevention

Prevention of opportunistic fungal pathogens such as aspergillosis in high-risk patients continues to be challenging. In the hospital setting, the current recommendation is the use of HEPA filtration as well as rooms with high-frequency air exchange and positive pressure.

Although in clinical practice some physicians use antifungal agents with *Aspergillus* activity as primary prophylaxis agents, there are no current studies or recommendations to promote this practice on a routine basis.

However, in certain situations antifugal agents are currently used as secondary prophylaxis. For instance, patients with a prior diagnosis of invasive aspergillosis who are going to undergo stem cell transplantation, solid organ transplantation, or a period of prolonged granulocytopenia and immunosuppression, should receive suppressive prophylaxis with either voriconazole 4 mg/kg b.i.d., itraconazole 300 mg b.i.d., or amphotericin B 1 mg/kg/d.

Suggested Readings

Caillot D, Couaillier JF, Bernard A, et al: Increasing volume and change characteristics of invasive pulmonary aspergillosis on sequential thoracic computed tomography scans in patients with neutropenia. *J Clin Oncol* 2001;19:253-259.

Herbrecht R, Denning DW, Patterson TF, et al: Voriconazole versus amphotericin B for primary therapy of invasive Aspergillosis. *N Engl J Med* 2002;347:408-415.

Mukherjee PK, Sheehan DJ, Hitchcock CA, et al: Combination treatment of invasive fungal infections. *Clin Microbiol Rev* 2005;18: 163-194.

Patterson TF: Aspergillosis. In: Dismukes WE, Pappas PG, Sobel JD, eds. *Clinical Mycology,* Oxford University Press, New York, 2003, pp 221-240.

Patterson TF: Aspergillus species. In: Mandell GL, Bennett JE, and Dolin R, eds. *Principles and Practice of Infectious Diseases*. Churchill Livingstone, Philadelphia, 2005, pp 2958-2972.

Patterson TF, Kirkpatrick WR, White M, et al: Invasive aspergillosis; disease spectrum, treatment practices, and outcomes. *Medicine* 2000;79:250-260.

Walsh TJ, Anaissie EJ, Denning DW, et al: Treatment of aspergillosis: clinical practice guidelines of the Infectious Diseases Society of America. *Clin Infect Dis* 2008;46:327-360.

Chapter 14

Zygomycosis (Mucormycosis, Phycomycosis)

Zygomycosis is an infection caused by the fungi of the orders Mucorales and Entomophthorales. These organisms are ubiquitous and generally saprophytic, rarely causing disease in the immunocompetent host, but are the third most frequent cause of invasive fungal infection in immunocompromised patients. The agents of zygomycosis are commonly found in the environment on fruit, bread, and soil. The organisms are common components of decaying organic debris.

The most common agent of zygomycosis (mucormycosis) is *Rhizopus arrhizus* (*Rhizopus oryzae*). The infection produced by zygomycosis agents is acute and rapidly fatal, despite early diagnosis and treatment. These organisms tend to invade major blood vessels, with ensuing ischemia, necrosis, and infarction of adjacent tissues and the production of black pus. Particularly at risk are granulocytopenic and acidotic patients. Fungi in the Zygomycetes class, for unknown reasons, tend to affect acidotic patients, particularly diabetic patients, but they have also been known to infect patients with acidosis secondary to renal insufficiency, diarrhea, and aspirin intake. Additional risk factors include glucocorticoid therapy, deferoxamine (Desferal®) therapy, and previous splenectomy. Recently, there appears to be a reported increase in mucormycosis among patients undergoing hematopoietic stem cell transplant. The etiology of this increase in unknown, although use of antifungal prophylaxis or therapy with either itraconazole (Sporanox®) or voriconazole (Vfend®) has been suggested.

Clinical Presentation

There are five major clinical forms of zygomycosis: (1) rhinocerebral, (2) pulmonary, (3) abdominal-pelvic and gastric (gastrointestinal), (4) primary cutaneous, and (5) disseminated.

Rhinocerebral Zygomycosis

The most frequently encountered form of infection is seen primarily in the acidotic, diabetic patient. The characteristic presentation generally involves the nose, followed by the eye, the brain, and, occasionally, the meninges.

Manifestations may include fever, unilateral facial pain, headaches, nasal congestion, epistaxis, visual disturbances, and lethargy. On physical examination there is periorbital cellulitis, proptosis, and loss of extraocular muscle movement. These lesions are frequently accompanied by cranial nerve palsy of the second, third, fourth, and sixth nerves. Additionally, black necrotic lesions are generally seen on the hard palate or nasal mucosa of these patients.

Differential diagnosis includes aspergillosis of the nasal cavity and sinuses, infections caused by *Scedosporium apiospermum* (*Pseudallescheria boydii*) and other filamentous molds, cavernous sinus thrombosis, bacterial sinusitis, and periorbital cellulitis.

Pulmonary Zygomycosis

Primary pulmonary zygomycosis occurs in patients with hematologic cancer or profound neutropenia and in those who have been on steroid therapy. The manifestations include fever, a productive cough with hemoptysis, chest pain, and increasing shortness of breath. Patients may also have a pleuritic rub and rhonchi over affected areas.

Differential diagnosis includes pulmonary aspergillosis, pulmonary infection with *S apiospermum* (*P boydii*) and other filamentous molds, and pulmonary infections caused by *Pseudomonas aeruginosa*.

Gastrointestinal Zygomycosis

Gastrointestinal zygomycosis usually results from ingestion of the organism by patients who are malnourished or have renal failure, and it produces necrotic ulcerations with ischemia and gangrene of the stomach and colon. The manifestations include fever, abdominal pain/distention, dyspepsia, nausea/vomiting, diarrhea, and, occasionally, hematochezia. On physical examination, there are decreased bowel sounds with guarding or rebound tenderness and localized-to-diffuse abdominal tenderness.

Differential diagnosis includes peptic ulcer disease, esophageal reflux disease, gastrointestinal carcinoma, gastrointestinal infection with *Aspergillus* or other filamentous molds, and mesenteric ischemia.

Cutaneous Zygomycosis

Cutaneous zygomycosis may be primary or secondary. Primary infection is usually caused by the direct inoculation of the organism into disrupted integument and has been associated with use of Elastoplast® bandages over biopsy sites or with burn patients with prior colonization. Secondary cutaneous infection is generally seen with widely disseminated zygomycosis as a consequence of hematogenous seeding. Manifestations may include a history of local trauma and a painful area. On physical examination, the skin lesions are generally single, beginning with induration and erythema and gradually developing into a necrotic ulcer with a characteristic dark central area. The margins of the ulcer tend to be sharply demarcated.

Differential diagnosis includes ecthyma gangrenosum, cutaneous aspergillosis, and cutaneous infections with other molds.

Disseminated Zygomycosis

Disseminated zygomycosis is seen in patients with hematologic cancers during neutropenia. It begins in the lungs and spreads to the central nervous system (CNS), producing infarction, necrosis, and abscess formation. It also disseminates to the liver, spleen, kidney, heart, and skin. The infection begins with the inhalation of conidia into the respiratory tract and subsequently spreads hematogenously throughout the body.

Clinical manifestations include headaches, fever, visual disturbances, and changes in mental status with lethargy, obtundation and coma, occasionally with a sudden onset of focal neurologic deficits. Necrotic ulcerations of the respiratory tract mucosa or the skin are not uncommon.

Differential diagnosis includes disseminated aspergillosis, nocardiosis, cryptococcosis, toxoplasmosis, lymphoma or cancer of the CNS, and bacterial brain abscess.

Diagnosis

Unfortunately, laboratory studies are nonspecific. The diagnosis relies on a high index of suspicion in a host with appropriate risk factors and evidence of tissue invasion with the characteristic appearance of broad, nonseptate hyphae with right-angle branches. There are no serologic tests available, and the blood cultures have no benefit.

In rhinocerebral zygomycosis, scrapings of the discharge may be examined with potassium hydroxide (KOH) to reveal broad, irregularly shaped hyphae with right-angle branching. Fungal stains of biopsy material obtained from affected tissue remain the mainstay for a definitive diagnosis. Fungal culture of biopsy tissue may also be helpful but is frequently negative, despite positive histopathology. In fact, fungal cultures are only positive in 15% to 25% of cases.

In pulmonary zygomycosis, sputum smears and cultures are rarely helpful. A lung tissue biopsy is needed for a definitive diagnosis.

In most cases of gastrointestinal zygomycosis, the diagnosis is made at surgery or postmortem examination. Fungal stains and cultures of biopsy material are needed for a definitive diagnosis.

Fungal stains and cultures of a skin biopsy are also necessary for a definitive diagnosis of cutaneous zygomycosis.

In disseminated zygomycosis, blood cultures are of no benefit. Fungal stains and cultures of affected tissue are needed, along with histopathologic identification of the fungus.

If CNS abnormalities are present, brain biopsy may be beneficial, along with analysis of the cerebrospinal fluid, although findings are nonspecific, even in the presence of brain involvement. Colony-stimulating factor abnormalities include a slightly increased opening pressure, modest pleocytosis with a predominance of polymorphonuclear cells, and mild protein elevation. Hypoglycorrhachia is unusual. Occasionally, erythrocytosis is detected. Fungal stains and cultures are rarely, if ever, positive.

On histopathology, fixed tissue can be stained with hematoxylin and eosin (H&E) and may demonstrate fungal hyphae using Grocott's methenamine silver (GMS) stain or periodic acid-Schiff (PAS) stain. The classic appearance of the fungus is broad, nonseptate hyphae with acute-angle branching.

Imaging studies may provide additional information and assist with the diagnosis. In rhinocerebral zygomycosis, plain radiographs of sinuses and orbits may demonstrate sinus mucosal thickening, with or without air-fluid levels, but this is a nonspecific finding. Computed tomography (CT) scans with contrast or magnetic resonance imaging may show erosion or destruction of bone and sinuses and delineate the extent of the disease. In pulmonary zygomycosis, chest radiographs may show single or multiple large mass-like infiltrates, pulmonary nodules, or cavitary lesions. These lesions, however, are indistinguishable from aspergillosis. A CT scan with contrast may help delineate the extent of the disease. For gastrointestinal zygomycosis, abdominal radiographs may show air under the diaphragm if a perforation has occurred. Barium studies of the upper gastrointestinal tract or colon may demonstrate a filling defect or a mass-like effect suggestive of zygomycosis. In disseminated zygomycosis, a CT scan of the thorax and head may show invasive disease and delineate the extent of the disease. Additionally, a CT scan of the abdomen and pelvis may show infiltrative lesions in the liver, spleen, kidney, pancreas, stomach, and omentum.

Treatment

Successful treatment of zygomycosis requires a high index of clinical suspicion for an early diagnosis. Mortality rates as high as 85% have been documented. Treatment requires: (1) reversal of underlying condition, when possible; (2) wide and extensive surgical removal of the affected tissue, which frequently includes multiple operations; and (3) early antifungal therapy. Unfortunately, prospective randomized clinical trials have not been performed. Current recommendations include using high dose lipid preparations of amphotericin B at doses of 10 to 15 mg/kg/d (Abelcet®, AmBisome®). The optimal duration of therapy is unknown, but a total dose of 2 to 6 g has been used in some cases. Using this aggressive therapeutic approach, several authors have demonstrated slightly improved outcomes in their patients with rhinocerebral zygomycosis, the most fulminant form of the disease, but the prognosis with gastrointestinal zygomycosis remains poor. When invasive zygomycosis complicates peptic ulcer disease without severe immunosuppression, surgical resection is often curative.

The mainstay of treatment, however, is still early and aggressive surgical debridement of affected tissue. Without early and aggressive therapy, zygomycosis is almost always fatal. An effort should be made to attempt to remove as much devitalized tissue as possible, and wide surgical debridement should be considered whenever feasible. Consultations may be necessary with specialists in infectious diseases, surgery, otorhinolaryngology, gastroenterology, pulmonary medicine, ophthalmology, and neurosurgery.

Additionally, one of the new triazoles, posaconazole (Noxafil®), has also demonstrated in vitro activity against many agents of zygomycosis. Voriconazole has not been shown to be active in vitro, and neither has the echinocandin group of antifungals.

Posaconazole in animal studies has been shown to be more effective than itraconazole, and as effective as the lipid preparations of amphotericin B in models of disseminated mucormycosis. Furthermore, there have been several reports describing the high overall success rate with posaconazole as a second-line agent in patients who are either intolerant of antifungals, or have refractory mucormycosis. Because there are no prospective trials, it is difficult to recommend posaconazole over the lipid preparations of amphotericin B as first-line therapy for mucormycosis, but posaconazole has certainly established itself as a primary alternative agent in patients failing amphotericin B or those who are intolerant of conventional antifungal therapy.

In addition to the antifungals, there are several reports of a successful outcome in patients given combination therapy with either amphotericin B or a liposomal derivative and granulocyte-colony stimulating factor.

Inpatient care is frequently prolonged because of the severe nature of the illness. Patients frequently undergo multiple surgical procedures in an attempt to eradicate all of the devitalized tissue, while the antifungals are generally provided parenterally for a prolonged time.

The overall prognosis of the infection depends on several factors, including the site of infection, the rapidity of diagnosis, and the type and severity of immunosuppression. The mortality rate is approximately 85% for patients with the rhinocerebral form of infection, and the overall mortality rate is approximately 50%. Factors in the elevated mortality rate include delays in diagnosis, poor antifungal activity of current compounds, and degree of immunosuppression. Thus, by the time the diagnosis is suspected or confirmed, the infection has frequently spread diffusely into the adjacent tissues and has produced extensive tissue destruction.

Suggested Readings

Garcia-Diaz JB, Palau L, Pankey GA: Resolution of rhinocerebral zygomycosis associated with adjuvant administration of granulocyte-macrophage colony-stimulating factor. *Clin Infect Dis* 2001;32: E145-E150.

Gaviria JM, Grohskopf LA, Barnes R, et al: Successful treatment of rhinocerebral zygomycosis: a combined-strategy approach. *Clin Infect Dis* 1999;28:160-161.

Ibrahim AS, Edwards JE, Filler SG: Zygomocoses. In: Dismukes WE, Pappas PG, Sobel JD, eds. *Clinical Mycology.* 1st ed. New York, NY, Oxford University Press, 2003, pp 241-251.

Kontoyiannis DP, Wessel VC, Bodey GP: Zygomycosis in the 1990s in a tertiary-care cancer center. *Clin Infect Dis* 2000;30:851-856.

Spellberg B, Edwards J, Ibrahim A: Novel perspectives on mucormycosis: pathophysiology, presentation, and management. *Clin Microbiol Rev* 2005;18:556-569.

Sugar AM: Agents of mucormycosis and related species. In: Mandell GL, Bennett JE, Dolin R, eds. *Principles and Practice of Infectious Diseases.* 6th ed. New York, NY, Churchill Livingstone, 2005, pp 2973-2984.

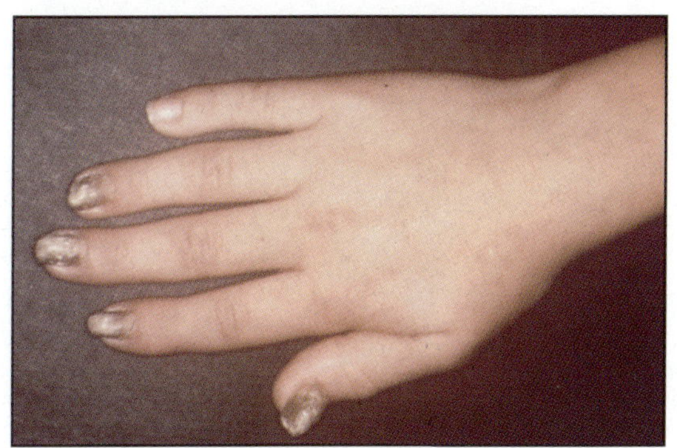

Figure 11-1: *Candida* onychomycosis.

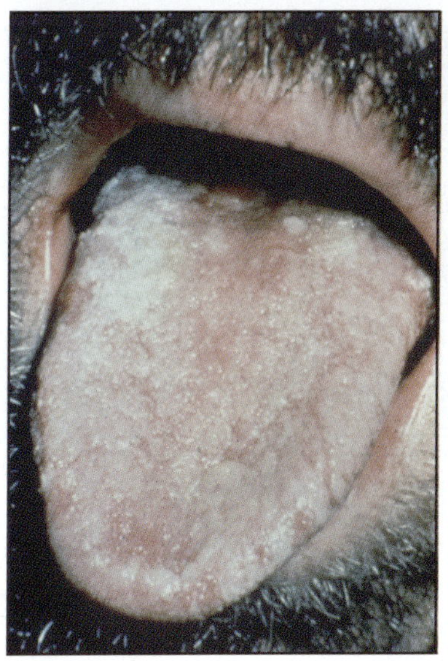

Figure 11-2: Oropharyngeal candidiasis (thrush).

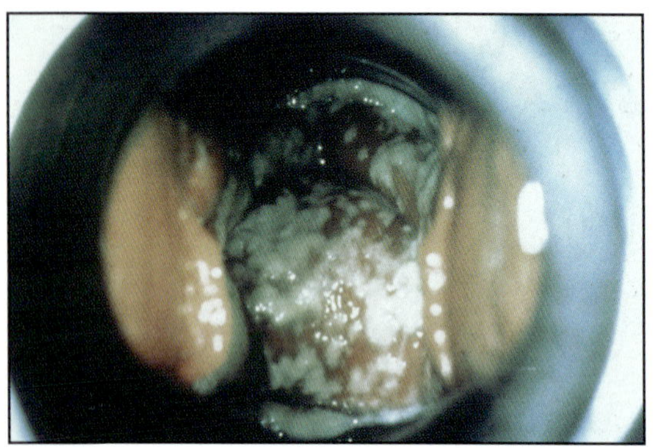

Figure 11-3: Vulvovaginal candidiasis.

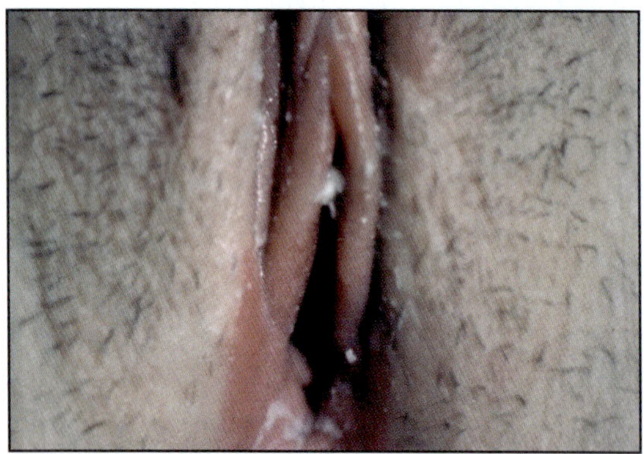

Figure 11-4: Vulvovaginal candidiasis.

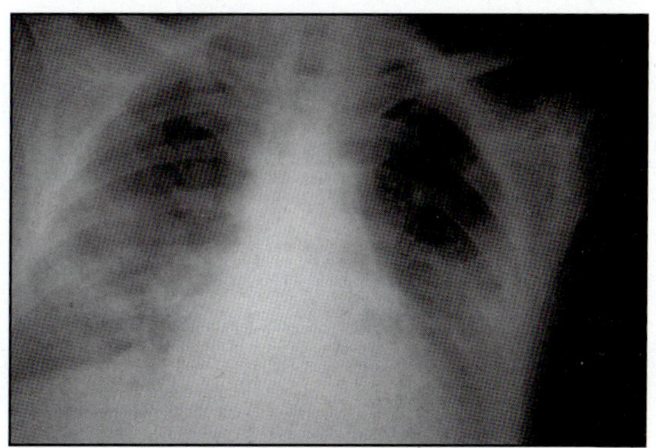

Figure 12-1: Pulmonary cryptococcosis.

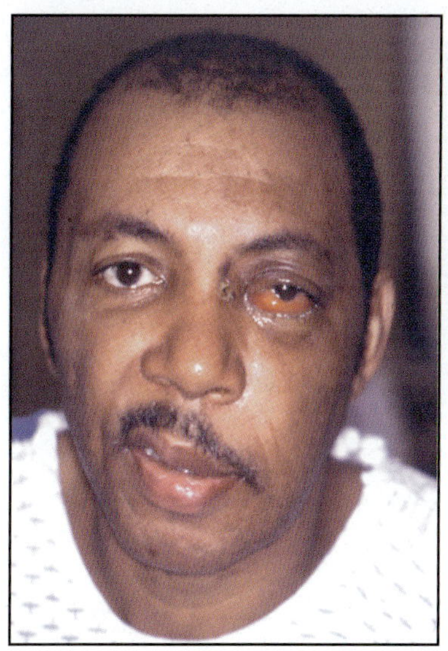

Figure 13-1: *Aspergillus* sinusitis.

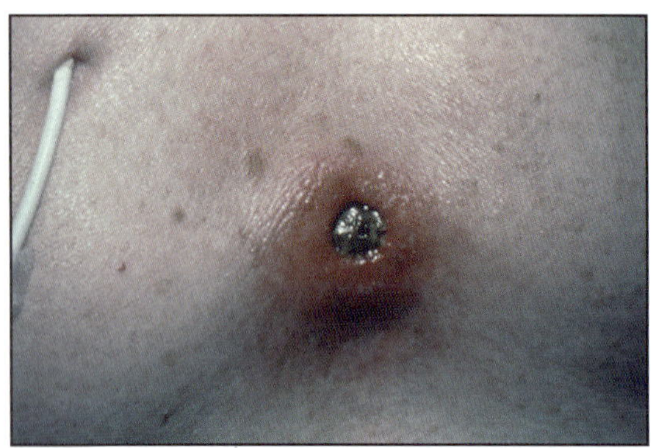

Figure 13-2: Cutaneous aspergillosis (disseminated disease).

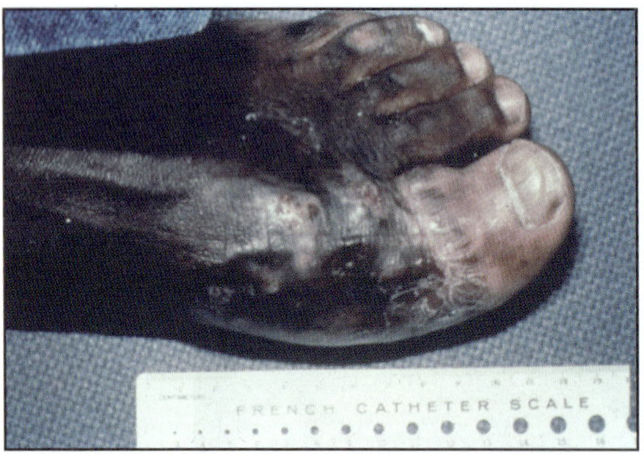

Figure 15-1: Mycetoma (Madura foot) caused by *Pseudallescheria boydii.*

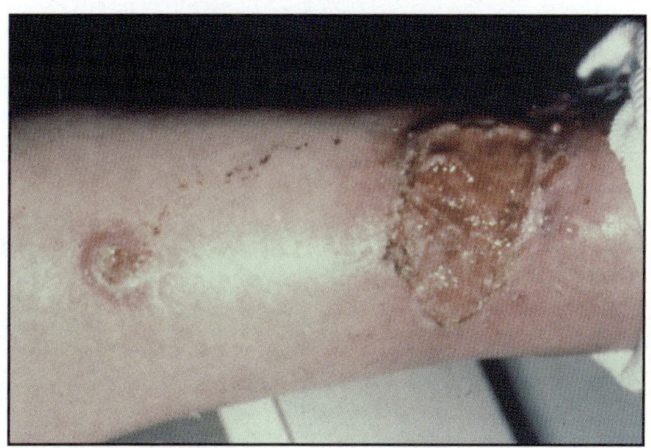

Figure 17-1: Ulcerative cutaneous blastomycosis.

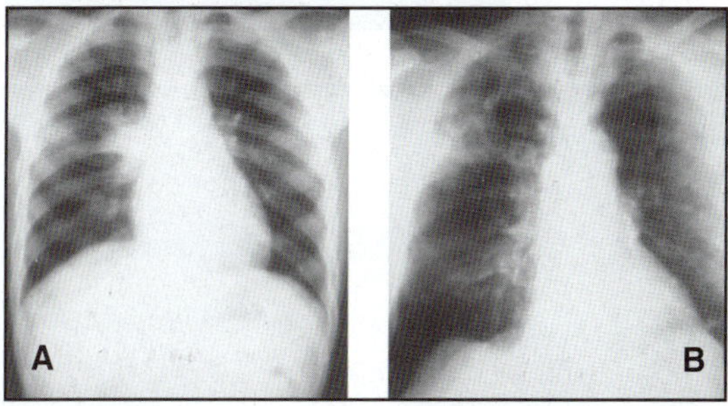

Figure 18-1: A. Acute pulmonary histoplasmosis; **B.** Chronic pulmonary histoplasmosis.

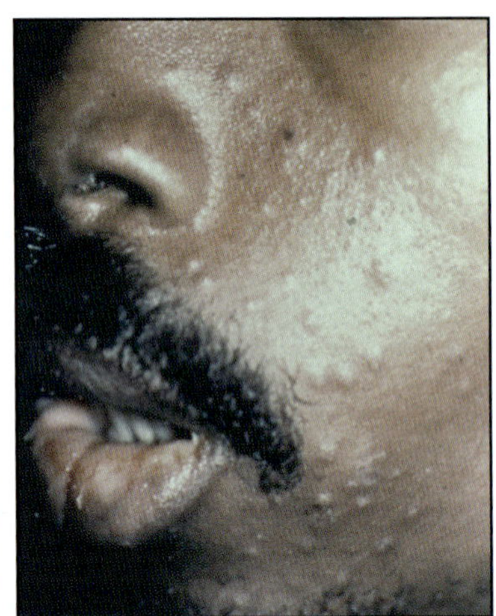

Figure 18-2: Disseminated histoplasmosis in patient with AIDS.

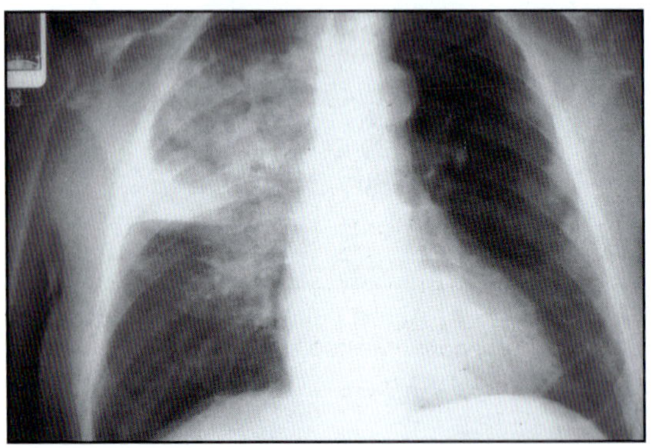

Figure 19-1: Acute pulmonary coccidioidomycosis.

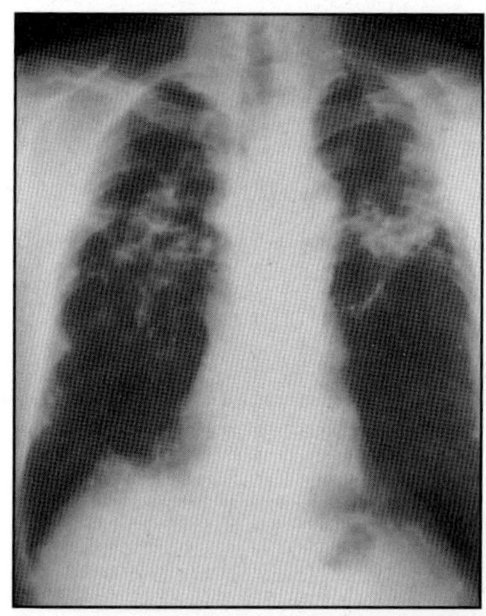

Figure 19-2: Chronic pulmonary coccidioidomycosis.

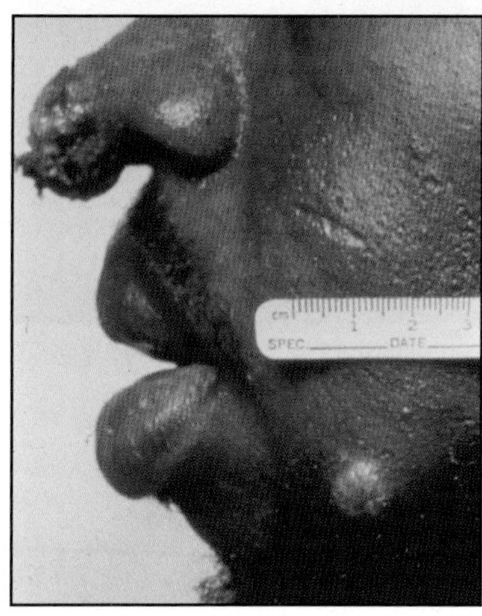

Figure 19-3: Cutaneous coccidioidomycosis (disseminated disease).

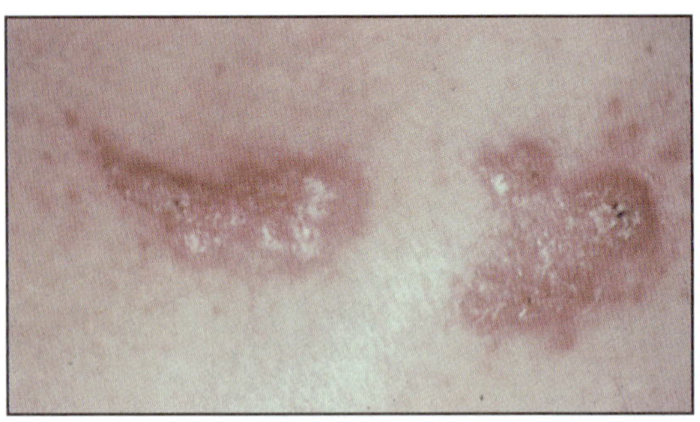

Figure 20-1: Fixed cutaneous sporotrichosis.

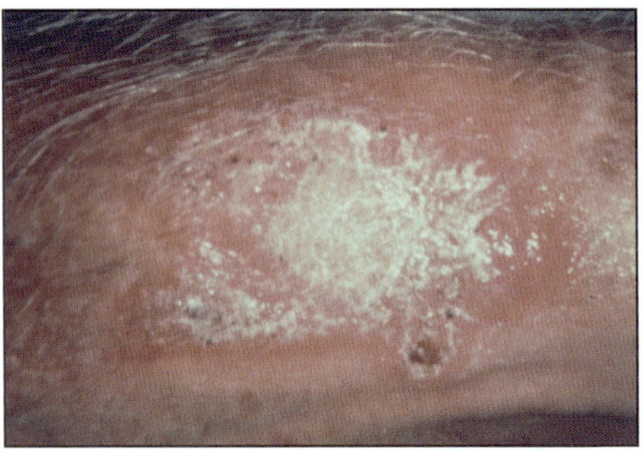

Figure 23-1: Chromoblastomycosis, tumorous lesion.

Chapter 15

Hyalohyphomycosis

Hyalohyphomycosis is a general term used to describe subcutaneous and systemic infections caused by nondematiaceous, hyaline molds. These molds have light-colored hyphal elements that may be branched, unbranched, or swollen (toruloid).

Hyalohyphomycosis encompasses an important and increasingly prevalent array of infections caused by saprobic fungi that are normally found in the soil but are emerging as a cause of opportunistic infection in the immunocompromised host. The most common etiologic agents in this group include *Fusarium moniliforme, Fusarium solani, Fusarium oxysporum, Chrysosporium* species, *Geotrichum candidum, Pseudallescheria boydii* (*Scedosporium apiospermum*), *Scopulariopsis acremonium, Scopulariopsis brevicaulis,* and *Paecilomyces* species (Table 15-1).

These fungi tend to invade the vascular system, as do *Aspergillus* species and agents in the Zygomycetes class. Accordingly, necrotic ulcers are usually accompanied by underlying thrombosis of adjacent blood vessels. Fungal culture is required for final identification of the infecting organism because hyalohyphomycosis has many clinical and histologic similarities to aspergillosis. Unlike *Aspergillus* species, several molds that cause hyalohyphomycosis, such as *Fusarium* species, are cultured from the blood in more than 50% of cases of disseminated disease. The appearance of new skin lesions that evolve

Table 15-1: Classification and Major Etiologic Agents of Hyalohyphomycosis

- *Acremonium* spp
  - *A alabamense*
  - *A falciforme*
  - *A kiliense*
  - *A roseogriseum*
- *Beauveria* spp
- *Chrysosporium* spp
- *Fusarium* spp
  - *F moniliforme*
  - *F oxysporum*
  - *F semitectum*
  - *F solani*
- *Geotrichum* spp
  - *G candidum*
  - *G klebhanii*
- *Microascus* spp
  - *M cinereus*
- *Paecilomyces* spp
  - *P lilacinus*
  - *P marquandii*
  - *P variotii*
  - *P viridis*
- *Penicillium* spp
  - *P argillaceae*
  - *P chrysogenum*
  - *P citrinum*
  - *P commune*
  - *P expansum*
  - *P marneffei*
  - *P spinulosum*
- *Pseudallescheria boydii (Scedosporium apiospermum)*
- *Schizophyllum commune*

from erythema to necrosis during the infection is also an important diagnostic clue to disseminated hyalohyphomycosis. Until recently, mortality rates associated with hyalohyphomycosis were higher than 95%, despite intensive antifungal therapy and surgical resection of the infected tissue. As with other fungal infections, the status of the host's defense mechanisms, the underlying disease, and the severity of dissemination are important factors in the final prognosis.

Fusarium Species

Fusarium species are the most common cause of invasive disease caused by hyalohyphomycosis. In many large cancer centers, they are the second or third most common cause of disseminated fungal infection in the immunocompromised host. *Fusarium* species are important plant pathogens and common soil fungi and are normally innocuous. Systemic disease from bloodstream dissemination is the most common form of fusariosis in humans. Although not yet as common as aspergillosis, fusariosis has epidemiologic characteristics, predisposing factors, clinical presentation, and histopathology similar to those of aspergillosis.

Epidemiology

Previously, systemic disease was observed following the ingestion of grain contaminated with *Fusarium* species and was associated with aplastic anemia and death. During World War II, one million people were poisoned by contaminated grain.

Today, the most common form of fusariosis involves blood stream dissemination and occurs in severely immunocompromised patients. These patients usually have an underlying hematologic malignancy and have received intensive chemotherapy accompanied by profound and prolonged neutropenia. The incidence of fusariosis in bone marrow transplant (BMT) recipients was reported to be 1% to 2% among patients undergoing allogeneic BMT and 0.2% among those undergoing autologous BMT. Major predisposing factors besides neutropenia include cytotoxic chemotherapy, BMT, severe burns, and high-dose corticosteroids. In the immunocompetent host, *Fusarium* species can produce localized disease of the nails (onychomycosis), skin, and subcutaneous tissues, usually by direct inoculation of infectious material. Occasionally, they may cause keratoconjunctivitis.

Although more than 50 species of *Fusarium* have been identified, only a few are known to produce infection in humans. The most common etiologic agent appears to be *F solani,* which is recovered in about 50% of cases, followed by *F moniliforme, F oxysporum,* and *F dimerum.* The small size of the conidia (spores) suggests that the portal of entry is primarily the respiratory tract, although entry through direct cutaneous inoculation or the gastrointestinal tract is possible.

Clinical Presentation

Fusariosis is frequently confused with aspergillosis because of the similarities in presenting manifestations and tissue histology.

Fusarium species can produce superficial, locally invasive, or disseminated infections. The syndromes associated with fusariosis include invasive sinusitis, rhinocerebral infection, endophthalmitis, cutaneous/soft tissue infection, osteomyelitis, pulmonary infection, and disseminated infection (Table 15-2).

Superficial fusariosis includes keratoconjunctivitis, onychomycosis, burn wound infections, surgical wound infections, otitis media, and otitis externa. *Fusarium* species are a common cause of keratoconjunctivitis, especially in the southern United States. Trauma and penetration of the cornea by soil or plants contaminated with fusaria is the usual route of infection, but keratoconjunctivitis secondary to use of contaminated contact lenses or steroid or antimicrobial eyedrops is also possible.

Locally invasive fusariosis includes osteomyelitis, septic arthritis, brain abscess, endophthalmitis, cystitis, peritonitis, pneumonia, and cutaneous and subcutaneous infections, including mycetoma. These infections occur primarily in immunocompromised hosts but can occur in immunocompetent hosts.

Disseminated fusariosis is seen primarily in the compromised host and has recently increased in incidence, especially in patients with hematologic malignancy. The characteristic syndrome seen in fusariosis is a persistent

Table 15-2: Syndromes Associated With *Fusarium* Infection

- Cutaneous infection (most common presentation [60% to 70%])
- Disseminated infection (second most common presentation [40% to 60%])
- Pulmonary infection (third most common presentation [20% to 30%])
- Subcutaneous infection
- Invasive sinusitis
- Rhinocerebral infection
- Endophthalmitis
- Keratoconjunctivitis
- Osteomyelitis
- Gastrointestinal infection

fever in a neutropenic host despite broad-spectrum antimicrobials. Approximately 60% to 75% of patients have painful skin lesions, which may be an early manifestation of disseminated disease. The lesions may be multiple erythematous subcutaneous nodules, ecthyma gangrenosum-like lesions, painful ulcerations with central infarction, or target lesions. Patients may also have nonspecific infiltrates or nodular lesions in the lung.

Diagnosis

Physicians caring for high-risk patients should have a high index of suspicion. Fusaria are the only opportunistic molds that can be easily recovered from the blood stream, and blood cultures are positive in 60% to 75% of patients with fusariosis. A skin biopsy should be obtained of any unusual skin lesion. However, although histopathology is helpful, microscopic findings are almost identical to those seen with infection by *Aspergillus* and *Scedosporium* species. The fungal culture is still the gold standard for a definitive diagnosis of fusariosis. *Fusarium* species are readily grown on standard fungal media such as Sabouraud dextrose agar.

Management

Patient survival is affected by the susceptibility of fusaria to antifungals. *Fusarium* isolates are frequently resistant to flucytosine (Ancobon®), many of the azoles, and, occasionally, amphotericin B (Amphocin®, Fungizone®). Early open-label clinical trials and compassionate clinical trials have demonstrated that the new US Food and Drug Administration (FDA)-approved triazole voriconazole (Vfend®) shows excellent activity against all *Fusarium* species. Voriconazole is approved at a dose of 6 mg/kg q 12 h for two doses followed by 4 mg/kg q 12 h for the management of fusariosis in patients unresponsive to or intolerant of other antifungal therapy. It demonstrates an increase in survival of approximately 40%, compared with the historical 10% success rate with amphotericin B products. Preliminary studies with the lipid preparations of amphotericin B (Abelcet®, AmBisome®, Amphotec®), which may be given in higher doses and have reduced toxicity compared to desoxycholate amphotericin B, have also shown some promise. A report of the successful treatment of a *Fusarium* infection in a severely immunocompromised child described evidence of synergy between amphotericin B and rifampin (Rifadin®, Rifadin®IV) used together with granulocyte transfusions. Posaconazole has also shown activity against *Fusarium*. In a study of 23 patients with fusariosis, posaconazole demonstrated an overall success rate of 48%.

Successful treatment depends on early diagnosis and treatment and the host's immune status. If possible, immunosuppression must be stopped or reduced by decreasing use of steroids, chemotherapy, or immunosuppressants and by correcting neutropenia with growth factors. Combination therapy with amphotericin B and caspofungin (Cancidas®) or voriconazole and caspofungin also demonstrates good synergistic activity in vitro. Prognosis remains poor with disseminated disease but correlates with resolution of neutropenia.

Pseudallescheria boydii (Scedosporium apiospermum)

Pseudallescheria boydii infections are usually seen in immunocompromised patients but may occur in immunocompetent hosts. The organism demonstrates uniform in vitro resistance to most antifungals, with the exception of miconazole (Micatin®, Monistat®) and the newer triazoles, voriconazole and posaconazole. Disseminated disease is frequently fatal and associated with central nervous system infection, but localized disease resulting from direct skin inoculation may be cured with medical and surgical therapy despite persistent immunosuppression.

This fungus is a saprobe that can be isolated from soil, animal manure, and polluted water. In the perfect state, it is known as *Pseudallescheria boydii*; in the imperfect state, it is known as *Scedosporium apiospermum*. *Pseudallescheria boydii* forms thin-walled cleistothecia and light brown, elliptical ascospores. Histologically, it resembles *Aspergillus fumigatus* and *Fusarium* species.

Patients become infected through inhalation of conidia or direct inoculation of the organism into the skin or subcutaneous tissues. Risk factors for infection are BMT, neutropenia, hematologic malignancy, solid organ transplant, and high-dose corticosteroids. *Pseudallescheria boydii* frequently produces superficial, subcutaneous, or locally invasive infection in immunocompetent hosts.

Clinical Manifestations

Pseudallescheria boydii produces a wide spectrum of syndromes that may mimic aspergillosis or fusariosis. These infections may be superficial, subcutaneous, locally invasive, or disseminated.

Superficial infections include keratoconjunctivitis, onychomycosis, burn wound infections, and otomycosis. As with *Fusarium* species, keratoconjunctivitis is most often the result of trauma to the cornea with direct inoculation of the organism, but it may be associated with contact lenses or steroid or antimicrobial eyedrops.

Locally invasive disease includes osteomyelitis, septic arthritis, brain abscess, endophthalmitis, cystitis, peritonitis, pulmonary infection, and cutaneous and subcutaneous infections, including mycetoma (Figure 15-1; see color plate insert). In the United States, *P boydii* is the most common cause of mycetoma. Pulmonary infections are the most frequent manifestation and include fungus balls, necrotizing pneumonia, solitary nodules, cavitary lesions, and empyema. Several cases of pneumonia have been reported in patients who have aspirated water during near-drowning episodes.

Disseminated disease generally occurs in severely immunocompromised hosts, especially in association with neutropenia and high-dose corticosteroids. In many cases, the mold disseminates hematogenously to other body sites. Brain abscess, meningitis, endophthalmitis, and endocarditis caused by *P boydii* have been documented.

Diagnosis

Pseudallescheria boydii is usually diagnosed on biopsy, although its pathologic characteristics resemble those of *Aspergillus* and *Fusarium* species. Because the organism can produce colonization without disease, its invasiveness should be demonstrated on histopathology. On culture, the colonies are brownish gray.

Management

Successful treatment depends on early diagnosis, initiation of appropriate antifungal therapy, and the host's immune status. If possible, immunosuppression must be stopped or reduced by decreasing corticosteroids, withholding chemotherapy or immunosuppressants, or correcting neutropenia with growth factors. Voriconazole (as monotherapy) is indicated for treatment of infections caused by *S apiospermum* in patients unresponsive to or intolerant of other antifungal therapy. Although not yet approved, successful outcomes have been reported in several cases of *S apiospermum* infection when posaconazole was used as salvage therapy. Combination antifungal therapy with either amphotericin B and caspofungin or voriconazole and caspofungin also shows some promise in vitro. In general, prognosis remains poor with disseminated disease but correlates with resolution of neutropenia.

Penicillium marneffei

Epidemiology

Penicillium marneffei is a dimorphic fungus endemic to Southeast Asia, where it is considered an opportunistic infection in patients with AIDS. Before AIDS emerged, it was a rare cause of fungal infections in immunocompetent and immunocompromised hosts in Southeast Asia. In Thailand, *P marneffei* is the third most common opportunistic pathogen in AIDS patients after *Mycobacterium tuberculosis* and *Cryptococcus neoformans.* Because of the increase in air travel, cases have now been reported worldwide.

Penicillium marneffei was initially recovered from bamboo rats in Vietnam; these rats are considered to be the most important reservoir of infection. Di Salvo et al were the first to describe the infection by natural cause in a missionary with Hodgkin's disease who had traveled to Southeast Asia. *Penicillium marneffei* was incidentally recovered from the spleen of the patient after an elective splenectomy.

Table 15-3: Risk Factors Associated With Penicilliosis

- Travel or living in Southeast Asia
- HIV infection with CD4 lymphocyte count <100 cells/mm^3
- Autoimmune hemolytic anemia
- Corticosteroids
- Hematologic/oncologic malignancy
- Renal transplant
- Systemic lupus erythematosus
- Malnutrition

The portal of entry is thought to be the respiratory or gastrointestinal tract. There is no direct evidence of disease transmission from rats to humans. Once the organism gains access, it proliferates within the histiocytes and disseminates throughout the body. The lung and liver appear to be the organs most frequently affected.

Although the disease affects both immunocompetent and immunocompromised hosts, most infections occur in immunocompromised hosts. The major risk factors for penicilliosis are listed in Table 15-3.

Clinical Manifestations

The clinical presentations of *P marneffei* infection are generally nonspecific, and the disease is generally more rapid and symptoms more acute in HIV-positive patients (Table 15-4). Symptoms may include fever, cough, generalized lymphadenopathy, hepatosplenomegaly, subcutaneous abscess, pulmonary infiltrates, and papular skin lesions that are usually diffuse and similar in appearance to molluscum contagiosum. Leukopenia and anemia are also common.

Table 15-4: Clinical Manifestations of Penicilliosis

- Fever
- Anemia
- Weight loss
- Skin lesions
- Fungemia
- Lymphadenopathy
- Cough
- Hepatomegaly
- Diarrhea
- Splenomegaly
- Pericarditis
- Arthritis
- Osteolytic lesions

Diagnosis

HIV-positive patients who live in or have traveled to an endemic area and who present with the above symptoms should be evaluated for penicilliosis. An early presumptive diagnosis can be made by microscopic examination of peripheral blood smears or fluid obtained from skin lesions, using Giemsa or Wright's stain. However, a skin biopsy and culture should be performed for a definitive diagnosis. On histopathologic stain, the yeast cells are best visualized by Gomori's methenamine silver (GMS) stain or periodic acid-Schiff (PAS) stain of tissues. They stain poorly with hematoxylin-eosin (H&E) stain.

15

On culture, *P marneffei* grows as a mold at 25°C and as a yeast at 37°C. Culture positivity may be obtained from a variety of sites. Histopathology reveals small, oval, yeast-like structures and long, tubular, sausage-like forms that grow intracellularly in histiocytes and resemble *Histoplasma capsulatum.*

Management

Without antifungal therapy, *P marneffei* infection is lethal. Recommended antifungal therapy includes initial therapy with intravenous amphotericin B 0.6 mg/kg/d for 2 weeks, followed by a switch to oral itraconazole (Sporanox®) 400 mg/d for 10 weeks. This combination therapy has a survival rate of more than 90% in HIV-positive patients. Approximately 25% of patients relapse within 6 months after completion of therapy. Thus, for patients with HIV infection and penicilliosis, secondary prophylaxis with oral itraconazole 200 mg/d for life is recommended. Use of azole antifungals alone as primary therapy has a success rate of 75% with itraconazole and 36% with fluconazole (Diflucan®).

In vitro susceptibility studies show that *P marneffei* is susceptible to ketoconazole (Nizoral®), itraconazole, miconazole, and voriconazole; has variable minimum inhibitory concentrations to amphotericin B; and is resistant to fluconazole.

Suggested Readings

Deng Z, Ribas JL, Gibson DW, et al: Infections caused by *Penicillium marneffei* in China and Southeast Asia: review of eighteen published cases and report of four more Chinese cases. *Rev Infect Dis* 1988;10:640-652.

Hospenthal DR: Uncommon fungi. In: Mandell GL, Bennett JE, Dolin R, eds. *Principles and Practice of Infectious Diseases*. 6th ed. New York, NY, Churchill Livingstone, 2005, pp 3068-3079.

Imwidthaya P, Thipsuvan K, Chaiprasert A, et al: *Penicillium marneffei*: types and drug susceptibility. *Mycopathologia* 2001;149: 109-115.

Nelson KE, Sirisanthana T: Penicilliosis. In: Dismukes WE, Pappas PG, Sobel JD, eds. *Clinical Mycology*. 1st ed. New York, NY, Oxford University Press, 2003, pp 355-364.

Ponton J, Ruchel R, Clemons KV, et al: Emerging pathogens. *Med Mycol* 2000;38:225-236.

Rinaldi MG: Emerging opportunists. *Infect Dis Clin North Am* 1989; 3:65-76.

Sirisanthana T: *Penicillium marneffei* infection in patients with AIDS. *Emerg Infect Dis* 2001;7:561.

Torres HA, Kontoyiannis DP: Hyalohyphomycosis. In: *Clinical Mycology*. 1st ed. New York, NY, Oxford University Press, 2003, pp 252-270.

Chapter 16

Phaeohyphomycosis

Phaeohyphomycosis is a general term for infections caused by dematiaceous (dark-walled) fungi. All dematiaceous fungi, on culture, have melanin-like pigment in the walls of their hyphae and/or conidia (spores). They can form yeast-like cells that are solitary or in short chains or hyphae that are septate, often irregularly swollen (toruloid), branched, or unbranched. They are normally associated with soil or vegetative matter. There are approximately 71 species in 39 genera. The most common etiologic agents in this group include *Bipolaris spicifera, Bipolaris hawaiiensis, Cladophialophora bantiana, Cladosporium cladosporioides, Curvularia geniculata, Exophiala jeanselmei, Phialophora parasitica,* and *Wangiella dermatitidis* (Table 16-1). Dematiaceous fungi are found worldwide in tropical, subtropical, and temperate climates. Most species are opportunistic pathogens, although some may be true pathogens.

The characteristic common to all dematiaceous fungi is the presence of melanin in the cell wall. Melanin has been shown by several investigators to be a virulence factor in several different fungi, such as *Cryptococcus neoformans* and *W dermatitidis*. It may confer a protective effect on the fungal cell by scavenging free radicals and hypochlorite produced by phagocytic cells that would kill most organisms. It may also bind to hydrolytic enzymes, thereby preventing their action on the plasma membrane.

Table 16-1: Classification of Phaeohyphomycosis and Etiologic Agents

Superficial Phaeohyphomycosis

- *Hortaea werneckii* (Syn: *Exophiala werneckii*)
- *Stenella araguata*

Cutaneous and Corneal Phaeohyphomycosis

- Dermatomycosis
  - *Alternaria* spp
  - *Scytalidium dimidiatum*
- Mycotic keratitis
  - *Botryodiplodia theobromae*
  - *Curvularia geniculata*
  - *Curvularia lunata*
  - *Curvularia senegalensis*
  - *Exophiala jeanselmei*
  - *Exserohilum rostratum* (Syn: *Drechslera rostrata*)
- Onychomycosis
  - *B theobromae*
  - *Phyllosticta* spp
  - *S dimidiatum*

Subcutaneous Phaeohyphomycosis

- *Alternaria alternata*
- *Bipolaris spicifera* (Syn: *Drechslera spicifera*)
- *Cladophialophora bantiana*
- *E jeanselmei*
- *Exophiala moniliae*
- *Exophiala spinifera*
- *Phialophora bubakii*
- *Phialophora parasitica*
- *Phialophora repens*
- *Phialophora richardsiae*
- *Phialophora verrucosa*
- *Scytalidium lignicola*
- *Wangiella dermatitidis*

Systemic Phaeohyphomycosis

- *Bipolaris* spp
    - *B hawaiiensis* (Syn: *Drechslera hawaiiensis*)
    - *B spicifera*
- *C bantiana*
- *Cladosporium cladosporioides*
- *C geniculata*
- *Curvularia pallescens*
- *Dissitimurus exedrus*
- *E jeanselmei*
- *W dermatitidis*

Classification

Phaeohyphomycosis can be classified by the region of the body in which the infection occurs: superficial, cutaneous, subcutaneous, and systemic.

Superficial infections are confined to the stratum corneum with minimal tissue response. If the hair is involved, the fungi grow superficially around the hair shaft with little damage to the hair. An example of this type of infection is black piedra (*Piedraia hortae*).

Cutaneous infections include infection of keratinized tissues, but they differ in the amount of tissue damage and the degree of host response. Nonliving tissue layers are usually involved and often exhibit extensive tissue destruction. Dermatomycosis, mycotic keratitis, and onychomycosis are examples of this type of infection.

Subcutaneous phaeohyphomycosis encompasses a group of infections that result from the traumatic implantation of the etiologic agent into the subcutaneous tissues. The lesions generally remain localized and form abscesses.

Systemic phaeohyphomycosis almost invariably occurs in the immunocompromised host. Most cases begin in the lungs and spread to other tissues by hematogenous dissemination. These infections, especially those involving the brain, have a grave prognosis. For example, *C bantiana* frequently invades the central nervous system (CNS). Infections with this organism frequently manifest as chronic headache followed by fever and focal neurologic defects. Occasionally, *C bantiana* produces localized pulmonary infection.

Immunocompromised patients, especially patients with neutropenia; bone marrow and solid organ transplant recipients; and HIV-positive patients are most at risk for phaeohyphomycosis. Immunocompetent hosts are occasionally infected. The primary routes of infection are direct traumatic implantation of the etiologic agent and inhalation of conidia.

Clinical Manifestations

Cutaneous infections include dermatomycosis, mycotic keratitis, and onychomycosis. Dermatomycosis differs from dermatophytosis in that the etiologic agents are dematiaceous fungi and not dermatophytes. The clinical presentations of both mycoses are very similar. Mycotic keratitis usually occurs secondary to implantation of the fungus during trauma or surgery to the eye. Most lesions present as pearly-gray fluffy exudates that precede superficial corneal ulcerations. Onychomycosis can be caused by any of the dematiaceous molds. Onychomycosis caused by these molds is similar in appearance to that caused by dermatophytes. However, the nail may have a dark pigmentation, which reflects the deposition of melanin pigment from the dematiaceous mold.

Subcutaneous infections are solitary cysts. These lesions are found at trauma sites and are frequently present for several months before diagnosis. There are usually no systemic signs or symptoms of infection. The nodules originate at the site of implantation. Purulent material may be found in the necrotic center in many lesions. On histopathology, there is a low-grade, localized, inflammatory response. Often, the organisms can be identified and cultured from examination of purulent exudates. The most commonly identified agents include *E jeanselmei, W dermatitidis, Bipolaris* species and *Phialophora* species.

Systemic disease includes a wide spectrum of infections and tissue invasions and primarily affects immunocompromised hosts. It may involve invasion of a single organ or disseminated infection. The portal of entry for the etiologic agent is usually the respiratory tract. Inhalation of conidia is followed by widespread dissemination throughout the body. The most frequently identified positive sites of infection are the blood (>50%), lung, heart, skin, brain, and kidneys.

Fungal sinusitis may be an allergic process that produces eosinophil-laden allergic mucin without tissue invasion or localized invasive disease. It may extend into the orbits or the cerebrum. Optic nerve involvement is rare.

Fungal pneumonia (most often caused by *B spicifera*) is another form of systemic infection. It is generally associated with chronic pulmonary infiltrates and relatively few constitutional symptoms. As with all types of phaeohyphomycosis, it occurs most often in severely compromised hosts.

Central nervous system infection is a severe form of systemic disease and is one of the most frequent manifestations of phaeohyphomycosis. *Cladophialophora bantiana,* which commonly infects the brain and meninges, is the agent most often associated with CNS infection. Patients generally have severe headaches, nausea, vomiting, and fever associated with altered mental status, seizures, and nuchal rigidity. Single or multiple lesions may be seen in images of the brain.

Disseminated infection frequently presents with fever, ulcerative skin lesions, cough, and shortness of breath. The overall mortality rate is about 79%; however, it is directly dependent on the site of infection and the degree of immunosuppression. The presence of neutropenia is also directly related to the mortality rate. The mortality rate in patients who do not recover from neutropenia is 100%.

Diagnosis

Diagnosis is generally confirmed by histopathologic examination of affected tissues when dematiaceous fungal elements are found in aspirated discharge of infected tissue, skin scrapings, or tissue biopsy. Fungal elements may be yeastlike and are usually positive for melanin by Masson-Fontana stain. Blood cultures are positive in approximately 50% of patients with disseminated disease. *Scedosporium prolificans* is the most common cause of phaeohyphomycosis. Serologic tests are not available.

Management

Surgical resection is often required for cure and is usually followed by administration of intravenous amphotericin B (Amphocin®, Fungizone®) or itraconazole (Sporanox®). The role of amphotericin B is controversial because of recent reports of poor in vitro activity. Clinical response has also been poor (23%) in patients treated with amphotericin B. However, no single antifungal agent has been associated with improved outcome.

Survival has been correlated with surgical removal of the lesions with or without antifungal therapy. One patient with disseminated *P parasitica* infection improved with terbinafine (Lamisil®), an oral allylamine. In vitro susceptibility assays also reveal considerable activity with itraconazole, voriconazole (Vfend®), and posaconazole. The echinocandins caspofungin (Cancidas®), micafungin (Mycamine®), and anidulafungin (Eraxis™) have also demonstrated in vitro activity against some dematiaceous fungi. Voriconazole and posaconazole have also demonstrated some clinical efficacy as described in several case reports.

Suggested Readings

Adam RD, Paquin ML, Petersen EA, et al: Phaeohyphomycosis caused by the fungal genera *Bipolaris* and *Exserohilum*. A report of 9 cases and review of the literature. *Medicine (Baltimore)* 1986;65:203-217.

Fader RC, McGinnis MR: Infections caused by dematiaceous fungi: chromoblastomycosis and phaeohyphomycosis. *Infect Dis Clin North Am* 1988;2:925-938.

Hospenthal DR: Uncommon fungi. In: Mandell GL, Bennett JE, Dolin R, eds. *Principles and Practice of Infectious Diseases.* 6th ed. New York, NY, Churchill Livingstone, 2005, pp 3068-3079.

Perfect JR, Schell WA, Cox GM: Phaeohyphomycoses. In: Dismukes WE, Pappas PG, Sobel JD, eds. *Clinical Mycosis.* 1st ed. New York, NY, Oxford University Press, 2003, pp 271-282.

Pritchard RC, Muir DB: Black fungi: a survey of dematiaceous hyphomycetes from clinical specimens identified over a five year period in a reference laboratory. *Pathology* 1987;19:281-284.

Chapter 17

Blastomycosis

Blastomyces dermatitidis is a dimorphic, round, budding yeast with daughter cells that form a bud with a broad base. Blastomycosis is generally an infection of the immunocompetent host, although it also occurs in the compromised host. *Blastomyces dermatitidis* is known to cause epidemics of infection and is endemic to certain geographical regions. While the yeast is reported worldwide, most cases are found along the Mississippi and Ohio River valleys. The precise ecology and epidemiology of this organism have been perplexing because of the difficulty in isolating it from the environment.

Blastomyces dermatitidis is the imperfect or asexual stage of *Ajellomyces dermatitidis*. The imperfect state exhibits dimorphism, found in mycelial form at room temperature and in yeast form at 37°C. Branching hyphae with conidiophores arise at right angles that produce single, terminal, round, or oval conidia. The conidia are infectious when the mycelia are disturbed. The yeast cells are multinucleated with 8 to 12 nuclei and reproduce by single buds with a broad base between parent and bud; the daughter cell is often as large as the mother cell before detachment. There are two serotypes.

Epidemiology

Endemic areas are the south central states, primarily those bordering the Mississippi and Ohio River basins, the Midwestern states, and states bordering the Great Lakes.

Table 17-1: Manifestations of Blastomycosis

- Pulmonary disease
  - Acute pneumonia
  - Chronic pneumonia
- Extrapulmonary disease
  - Osteomyelitis
  - Genitourinary infection
  - Central nervous system infection

The organism exists in wooded areas in warm, moist soil that is rich in organic debris, such as decaying vegetation or animal manure. Isolation of the fungus has also been documented from bodies of water, such as rivers, lakes, and ponds.

Pathogenesis

Infection occurs by inhalation of the conidia from the mycelial phase into the lung, followed by phagocytosis of the organism by bronchopulmonary mononuclear cells that produce a primary pulmonary infection. The extrapulmonary manifestations are the result of dissemination from the primary pulmonary infection via the lymphatics and the blood stream. The inflammatory response consists of clusters of polymorphonuclear leukocytes with noncaseous granulomas with epithelioid and giant cells. Despite a spontaneous resolution of fungal pneumonia in some cases, endogenous reactivation may occur at either pulmonary or extrapulmonary sites with or without previous therapy.

Manifestations

Blastomycosis is a systemic disease with a wide variety of pulmonary and extrapulmonary manifestations in about

60% of cases (Table 17-1). The extrapulmonary manifestations include cutaneous infections (the most common form of extrapulmonary infection), followed by bone and joint infections, genitourinary tract infections, and central nervous system infections.

Primary Pulmonary Blastomycosis

In most patients, the clinical presentation of blastomycosis is pneumonia. Primary lesions occur after the inhalation of the conidia into the respiratory tract, often mimicking tuberculosis or histoplasmosis. The incubation period varies between 21 and 100 days. Many patients are asymptomatic or have nonspecific symptoms with an abrupt onset of myalgias, arthralgias, fever, chills, transient pleuritic chest pain, and nonproductive cough.

Chest radiographs show alveolar or masslike infiltrates with lobar or segmental consolidation, primarily in the lower lobes. Occasionally, a miliary or reticulonodular pattern may be seen on chest radiograph. Afterward, the lesions may disappear with or without dissemination. The primary lung infection tends to heal with fibrosis and absorption. If the fungus spreads, it may lead to dissemination to skin and osseous structures.

Chronic or Recurrent Infection

This type of infection occurs when the primary pulmonary infection does not resolve. Blastomycosis is frequently diagnosed during this stage, when patients have chronic pneumonia with a productive cough, hemoptysis, weight loss, pleuritic chest pain, low-grade fever, and, occasionally, respiratory failure from miliary disease.

Chest radiograph during this stage shows upper lobe fibronodular infiltrates with or without cavitary lesions, mass lesions, miliary disease from hematogenous spread, diffuse pneumonitis, pleural thickening and pleural effusions, and pneumothorax.

Cutaneous Blastomycosis

Cutaneous blastomycosis is seen in 40% to 80% of cases, usually in conjunction with active pulmonary disease. It occurs after dissemination of the organisms from the respiratory tract. There are two types of lesions, the verrucous lesion and the ulcerative lesion. Verrucous lesions are seen on exposed areas and begin as small, papulopustular lesions that slowly spread to form a crusted, heaped-up lesion. Pathology reveals peripheral microabscesses with a purulent discharge when the eschar is removed. Ulcerative lesions start as pustules and spread as a superficial ulcer with slightly raised borders around a bed of red granulation tissue that bleeds easily (Figure 17-1; see color plate insert). These lesions may also occur on the mucosa of the nose, mouth, and pharynx.

The subcutaneous nodules are generally 'cold abscesses,' usually seen in conjunction with pulmonary and other extrapulmonary disease. Patients tend to be acutely ill with systemic symptoms. Rapid deterioration occurs unless treatment is started early.

Bone and Joint Blastomycosis

This is the second most frequently encountered extrapulmonary infection, occurring in 10% to 50% of patients, and is primarily seen in the long bones, vertebrae, pelvis, sacrum, skull, and ribs. The disease produces a well-circumscribed osteolytic lesion that is rarely associated with pain. It may also present with contiguous soft tissue abscesses or chronic draining sinuses. Biopsy of bone may show granulomas, suppuration, or necrosis. The radiographic appearance is indistinguishable from other fungal, bacterial, or neoplastic diseases.

Genitourinary Tract Blastomycosis

In about 30% of cases in men, the genitourinary tract is infected during widespread dissemination originating from the respiratory tract. The infection primarily involves the prostate and epididymis but may also spread to the testes. Urinalysis performed after prostatic massage will improve the detection of urinary infection.

Central Nervous System Infection

This infection is uncommon, occurring in 5% to 10% of cases of disseminated infection. The manifestations include brain abscesses or meningitis accompanied by headaches, seizures, confusion, coma, paraparesis, aphasia, and hemiparesis. It is generally a late infection and has fulminant symptoms of widely disseminated blastomycosis. Cerebrospinal fluid analysis usually does not reveal the organism, but the ventricular fluid has a higher yield.

Although most frequently found in the subcutaneous tissues, abscesses may also be found in the brain, skeletal system, prostate, myocardium, pericardium, orbit, sinuses, pituitary, and adrenal glands. The reticuloendothelial system has been involved with reports of lymph node, hepatic, or splenic infection.

Diagnosis

The diagnosis is made by direct examination of secretions, followed by culture. Cultures are positive in 2 to 4 weeks. Histopathology of infected tissues with fungal stains is also helpful. Serology is available, but it lacks sensitivity and specificity and so is not useful for diagnosing blastomycosis. The immunodiffusion assay has greater sensitivity and specificity and is positive in about 50% to 80% of cases. The enzyme-linked immunosorbent assay is also available. However, a negative test should never rule out infection, nor should a positive test be an indication to initiate therapy.

Skin testing with blastomycin is no better than serology as a diagnostic tool. This mycelial-phase antigen does not provide sufficient specificity and is no longer available clinically.

Table 17-2: Current Treatment Recommendations for Blastomycosis

Infection	Treatment
Pulmonary Disease	
Mild–to-moderate	Itraconazole 200-400 mg/d for 6–12 months
Severe—life threatening disease	Lipid amphotericin B 3-5 mg/kg/d or amphotericin B deoxycholate 0.7-1.0 mg/kg/d for 7-14 days; switch to itraconazole 400 mg/d for 6-12 months
Disseminated disease	
Mild-to-moderate	Itraconazole 200-400 mg/d for 6–12 months
Severe—life threatening disease	Lipid amphotericin B 3-5 mg/kg/d or amphotericin B deoxycholate 0.7-1.0 mg/kg/d for 7-14 days; switch to itraconazole 400 mg/d for 6-12 months
CNS disease	Lipid amphotericin B 5 mg/kg/d for 4-6 weeks; switch to itraconazole 600 mg/d, fluconazole 800 mg/d, or voriconazole 400-800 mg/d for12 months
Infection in immunocompromised host	Lipid amphotericin B 5 mg/kg/d for 7-14 days; followed by itraconazole 400 mg/d for at least 12 months. Consider life-long suppression if immunosuppression cannot be improved.

Management

Itraconazole (Sporanox®) 200–400 mg/d for 6–12 months is the standard of care for mild-to-moderate pulmonary infection and for mild-to-moderate disseminated infection. Amphotericin B deoxycholate 0.7–1.0 mg/kg/d or lipid amphotericin B 3–5 mg/kg/d is recommended for severe disease or CNS infection. The Infectious Diseases Society of America published clinical practice guidelines for the management of blastomycosis in June 2008 (Table 17-2).

Suggested Readings

Bradsher RW: Blastomycosis. In: Dismukes WF, Pappas PG, Sobel JD, eds. *Clinical Mycology.* 1st ed. New York, NY, Oxford University Press 2003, pp 229-310.

Chapman SW: Blastomyces dermatitidis. In: Mandell GL, Bennett JE, Dorlin R, eds. In: *Principles of Infectious Diseases.* 7th ed. New York, NY, Churchill Livingstone, 2005, pp 3026-3040.

Chapman SW, Bradsher RW Jr, Campbell GD Jr, et al: Practice guidelines for the management of patients with blastomycosis. Infectious Diseases Society of America. *Clin Infect Dis* 2000;30:679-683.

Chapman SW, Dismukes WE, Proia LA, et al: Clinical practice guidelines for the management of blastomycosis: 2008 update by the Infectious Diseases Society of America. *Clin Infect Dis* 2008; 46:1801-1812.

Klein BS, Vergeront JM, Davis JP: Epidemiologic aspects of blastomycosis, the enigmatic systemic mycosis. *Semin Respir Infect* 1986; 1:29-39.

Sarosi GA, Davies SF: Endemic mycosis complicating human immunodeficiency virus infection. *West J Med* 1996;164:335-340.

Chapter 18

Histoplasmosis

Histoplasma capsulatum is a dimorphic fungus with worldwide distribution. It is found primarily in the central regions of the United States, from the Gulf Coast to the Great Lakes. Histoplasmosis is the most common systemic endemic mycosis in the United States.

Histoplasma capsulatum is the imperfect state of a dimorphic fungus belonging to the Ascomycetes. The perfect state is called *Emmonsiella capsulata*. In its native habitat, the soil, it exists in a mycelial phase, but it converts to a yeast phase at 37°C. The mycelial form consists of septate branching hyphae with spores at lateral terminal positions. The spores, the infectious agent, are either microconidia or macroconidia. The yeast form is ovoid, and reproduction is by budding. In viable tissue, the organism is found almost entirely within the macrophages.

Epidemiology

The fungus grows readily in soil with a high nitrogen content, particularly soil enriched by bird and bat guano. It has been associated with blackbird roosts, pigeon roosts, chicken houses, and sites frequented by bats, such as caves, attics, old buildings, chimneys, decayed wood piles, and dead and hollow trees. In endemic areas, such places are most likely to be point sources. *Histoplasma capsulatum* spores are also found in soil in endemic areas. In some endemic areas, histoplasmosis is one of the most common opportunistic infections in patients with AIDS.

Although the fungus may be recovered worldwide, its greatest prevalence is in the temperate zones of the Americas. Moderate temperatures and shady areas make the river valleys of Ohio and Mississippi endemic areas. Inhabitants of these regions are probably repeatedly infected and are asymptomatic.

Pathogenesis

Spores are inhaled, reach the bronchioles or alveoli, and germinate after 48 to 72 hours, producing the yeast form of the fungus, which is promptly ingested by macrophages. The infected macrophages then migrate to mediastinal lymph nodes and the rest of the reticuloendothelial system (RES), primarily the spleen and liver. New focal infiltrates develop at these sites and are primarily prominent in mediastinal lymph nodes. Caseous lesions are encapsulated and eventually calcified. The usual infection is asymptomatic, and most patients will have small calcifications in the lung, lymph nodes, liver, and spleen. The immunity is primarily cell mediated. Moderate inhalation produces disease in 10 to 16 days. Heavy inhalation will result in symptomatic disease, even in fully immune people, although the incubation period is only 3 to 5 days and the illness is shorter in duration and less severe. In a small percentage of patients, a more severe form of progressive pulmonary infection or disseminated disease may occur. These patients tend to be infants with immature immune systems, patients with immunosuppression secondary to chemotherapy, patients on steroids, or patients with HIV infection.

Clinical Manifestations

The clinical syndromes associated with *H capsulatum* infection include (1) acute self-limited syndrome, (2) disseminated histoplasmosis, (3) chronic pulmonary histoplasmosis, (4) mediastinal granulomas, and (5) fibrosing mediastinitis (Table 18-1).

Table 18-1: Characteristic Clinical Presentation of Histoplasmosis

Acute respiratory symptoms	65.5%
Chronic pulmonary symptoms	8.4%
Disseminated infection	10.6%
Pericarditis	5.5%
Rheumatologic	6.0%
Asymptomatic	12.4%

Acute Pulmonary Histoplasmosis

The acute syndrome in the normal host is mild and self-limited. Manifestations include fever, headache, chills, nonproductive cough and pleuritic chest pain, malaise, anorexia, weight loss, myalgias, arthralgias, and fatigue in at least two thirds of patients. Patients frequently have a normal physical examination but may present with hepatosplenomegaly, adenopathy, and a variety of rashes. The most common rashes associated with the acute syndrome include erythema nodosum, erythema multiforme, and a diffuse maculopapular rash.

More than 75% of patients have a normal chest radiograph; some exhibit 2 cm clusters of small infiltrates, large hilar nodes, or mediastinal lymph nodes, with eventual calcifications or an occasional biliary pattern (Figure 18-1; see color plate insert). The large infiltrates leave caseous nodules that produce rounded 'buckshot' calcifications. Small pleural effusions occur in about 10% to 20% of acute infections. Although rare, massive effusions may signify erosion of a lymph node or parenchymal lesion into the pleural space. However, most pleural effusions are benign and heal spontaneously.

The duration of illness tends to be related to the severity of symptoms, with mild symptoms usually lasting 1 to 5 days, moderate symptoms 5 to 7 days, and severe manifestations 2 to 3 weeks. Because the disease is frequently self-limited, treatment with antifungals is unnecessary.

Rare Complications

Tracheal, bronchial, or esophageal obstruction. The obstructions are caused by marked enlargement of paratracheal lymph nodes, although they are not critical and usually subside spontaneously. Only occasionally will surgical excision of the obstruction be required.

Acute pericarditis. Acutely inflamed lymph nodes contiguous to the pericardium may induce an acute inflammatory reaction with fibrinous pericarditis but without penetration of a granulomatous adenitis. Cultures of the pericardial fluid and pericardium are negative. Rarely, granulomatous pericarditis may occur by softening and emptying of the lymph node contents into the pericardial sac. The acute pericarditis syndrome heals spontaneously, with fewer than 15% of patients developing constrictive pericarditis. However, approximately 25% of these patients may exhibit pericardial tamponade.

Mediastinal granuloma. This occurs when a group of large caseous lymph nodes, more often in the right paratracheal area, break down and become encapsulated into a single mass. Occasionally, large masses (~10 cm) invade vascular tissue, especially the superior vena cava, subsequently producing venous obstruction. No treatment is required in most cases; however, surgical removal is occasionally required to remove the obstruction.

Disseminated Histoplasmosis

Disseminated histoplasmosis is rare and potentially life threatening. Because it generally results from a defect in host immunity, it is regarded as an opportunistic infection. The groups at greatest risk include immunocompromised hosts, such as infants with immature immunity, HIV-positive patients, and patients with AIDS. Occasionally, a host with no known immune defects may develop this syndrome. The severity of disease depends on the degree of involvement of the RES and the underlying immune dysfunction.

The first syndrome is acute (infant-type), which has a high degree of RES involvement and is found predominantly in infants. Manifestations and the disease spectrum parallel the degree of diffuse involvement of the RES. In acute disseminated histoplasmosis, there is massive involvement of the RES with closely packed macrophages engorged with yeast forms. Fever is uniformly present, as is severe hepatosplenomegaly, generalized lymphadenopathy, weight loss, nausea, vomiting, and diarrhea. Frequently, superficial ulcerations of the oral mucosa are present.

The second form of infection is subacute or intermediate disseminated histoplasmosis. There is only moderate involvement of the RES with only a moderate degree of macrophage parasitization. Manifestations tend to be caused by the development of focal lesions in various organ systems, accompanied by fever, weight loss, and weakness. Approximately 25% of patients have some type of focal lesion. Gastrointestinal (GI) tract involvement is common, with associated ulcers of the ileum and colon, occasionally leading to obstruction, perforation, and peritonitis. Other forms of local invasion include adrenal gland invasion, endocarditis, meningitis, and focal cerebritis. Deep oropharyngeal ulcers with rolled edges occur in about 25% of patients, along with hepatosplenomegaly, which is almost always present. Autopsy studies reveal GI tract involvement in 70% of cases and oropharyngeal involvement in 67% of cases. Chest radiograph may rarely show interstitial pneumonitis. If the infection is untreated, it may be fatal within 10 to 12 months.

The third syndrome, chronic (adult-type) disseminated histoplasmosis, has the mildest degree of RES involvement and the mildest degree of macrophage parasitization. It is seen predominantly in adults. Manifestations in this syndrome are mild, chronic, and occasionally intermittent. Oropharyngeal ulcerations are the predominant findings and are caused by focal granulomatous lesions. Gradual weight loss, fatigue, and weakness are the most common complaints. Focal lesions producing meningitis, endocarditis, papular or plaque-like cutaneous lesions, and Addison's disease are also common. Frequently, tuberculoid granulomas are found on biopsy. Hepatosplenomegaly, intestinal ulceration, and interstitial pneumonitis are rare. Pancytopenia, caused by bone marrow suppression, is not uncommon. On chest radiograph, there is usually interstitial pneumonia that may be fatal in less than 4 weeks if untreated.

In patients with AIDS and disseminated histoplasmosis (Figure 18-2; see color plate insert), the syndrome is often acute and severe, with associated circulatory shock, respiratory failure, and disseminated intravascular coagulation present in 33% of cases. The oropharyngeal mucosa is rarely involved, and GI tract involvement is rare.

Chronic Pulmonary Histoplasmosis

Chronic pulmonary histoplasmosis is seen in normal immunity and takes advantage of structural defects of the lung to colonize abnormal pulmonary spaces caused by centrilobular and/or bullous emphysema. The parasitization causes a chronic destructive disease in the apical areas of the lungs (Figure 18-2; see color plate insert). Two types of lesions are associated with chronic pulmonary histoplasmosis—infected air spaces and pneumonic lesions. There are also two types of infected air spaces: infected centrilobular air space with small, rounded, fluid-filled spaces that are seen in the central lung zones, and large apical and subapical cavities representing preexisting bullous air spaces with a caseous lining and many organisms. The pneumonic lesions are segmental areas of interstitial pneumonitis. These areas have a tendency to develop central or scattered focal areas of coagulation-type necrosis.

There is possible vasculitis induced by ischemia, while organisms are rarely profound.

Manifestations frequently mimic pulmonary tuberculosis and include malaise, fever, chills, weight loss, productive mucoid cough with occasional hemoptysis, and pleuritic chest pain. Symptoms may persist for about 4 to 5 weeks.

Laboratory examinations include a histoplasmin skin test that is positive in >80% of patients and a complement fixation test that may be negative in about 25% of patients. Sputum smears with Wright's stain are positive in approximately 50% to 80% of patients, and sputum cultures are positive about 70% of the time, with higher rates in patients with cavitary disease. Laboratory studies may show anemia of chronic disease, leukocytosis, or lymphopenia and elevation in alkaline phosphatase.

On chest radiograph, pneumonic lesions are segmental or subsegmental, usually posterior laterally, and almost always limited to the apical posterior zones. The infection begins with an interstitial pneumonitis, followed by focal areas or large central area of necrosis. In cavitary disease, the thin-walled cavities tend to have fewer organisms and often heal without any form of therapy. The thick-walled cavities have greater numbers of organisms and do not heal if left untreated. Occasionally, there is increased fibrosis and enlargement with obstruction of normal tissue. This so-called 'marching cavity' is associated with increased fibrosis elsewhere in the lung.

Mediastinal Granulomas

Histoplasmosis may produce obstruction of major mediastinal structures because of large granuloma formation. The granulomas are the result of slow capsule formation around caseous lymph nodes. This results in an enlarging fibroma-like mass, occasionally up to 3 to 5 cm in diameter. These granulomas may compress the esophagus, superior vena cava, large airways, and pulmonary vessels. Occasionally, the granulomas may rupture into the esophagus, bronchus, or mediastinum. Calcifications or laminations of calcification are seen peripherally on chest radiograph, but they rarely produce significant tissue damage.

Fibrosing Mediastinitis

Mediastinal fibrosis consists of caseous lymph nodes associated with periadenitis and heals with fibrous encapsulation adhering to adjacent structures. It produces bronchial stenosis; occlusion of pulmonary arteries, veins, and the superior vena cava; and esophageal obstruction. Clinical manifestations vary, depending on the structure affected. The diagnosis is made on computed tomography of the chest.

Other Syndromes Associated With *Histoplasma capsulatum*

Broncholithiasis is pulmonary mediastinal calcification that may enlarge and form calcifications in the lung tissue or bronchial lymph nodes. Broncholiths eventually may soften and dissect into a bronchus, causing the expectoration of gritty material or small stones. Lithoptysis with or without hemoptysis and coughing paroxysms are the main findings. These episodes are benign events and rarely require any specific form of treatment.

Sinuses and fistulas are caused by caseous mediastinal lymph nodes that may occasionally soften and dissect into adjacent structures such as the bronchus, pericardium, or esophagus or, rarely, into two organs to cause a fistula. Bronchoesophageal fistulas are common and require corrective surgery.

Ocular histoplasmosis syndrome is seen in healthy, young adults. Organisms have rarely been found in the eyes. The manifestations include a triad of scattered, yellow, punched-out choroidal lesions, macular subretinal neovascular membranes, and peripapular atrophy, all without inflammatory signs. Vision improves spontaneously.

Diagnosis

The diagnosis of histoplasmosis depends on many factors, including type of infection, type of host, and source of infection. Diagnosis of disseminated disease depends on demonstration of the fungus in culture material from blood, urine, bone marrow, the liver, or other affected tissue. Frequently, organisms are found within well-formed granulomas and within oral ulcers. The histologic examination of Giemsa-stained sections may reveal small, yeast-like *H capsulatum* within lamina propria macrophages. Scrapings of oropharyngeal ulcerations are frequently positive on stains and always positive on biopsy. Liver biopsy is positive with either fungal stain or culture approximately 80% of the time.

Although cultures are frequently helpful, they are only positive in patients with chronic pulmonary histoplasmosis or disseminated histoplasmosis. Frequently, however, cultures may be the only way to establish infection. The specimens to culture include blood, using the lysis-centrifugation technique; sputum, using bronchoalveolar lavage; and bone marrow biopsy. Occasionally, cultures of urine, cerebrospinal fluid, lymph nodes, and oral lesions may be positive.

Skin Test

Histoplasmin test is not helpful and may boost subsequent complement fixation titers.

Serology

Complement fixation tests for the presence of serum antibodies to *H capsulatum*. Yeast-phase antigen is more sensitive than mycelial-phase titer of 1:32 or greater or fourfold increase. Immune diffusion is more specific but less sensitive than complement fixation. It measures two bands, M bands and H bands. Both bands are specific, but they occur infrequently. H bands alone are rare.

Table 18-2: Treatment of Histoplasmosis

Indicated	*Not Indicated*
• Disseminated	• Mediastinal fibrosis
• Chronic pulmonary	• Pulmonary
• Acute pulmonary with hypoxia	• Broncholithiasis
• Acute pulmonary >1 month	
• Severe	

Antigen Detection of Histoplasmosis

This is the most sensitive assay commercially available for the diagnosis of histoplasmosis. It detects a polysaccharide antigen of histoplasma in urine or serum. The test is now performed using an enzyme-linked immunosorbent assay (ELISA), which is equivalent to the prior radioimmunoassay detection test. The antigen sensitivity is approximately 90% in disseminated histoplasmosis, 40% in cavitary histoplasmosis, and 20% in acute pulmonary syndrome. The assay can also monitor for relapses, especially in immunocompromised patients with disseminated disease.

Treatment

Antifungal therapy is used for more severe cases of histoplasmosis (Table 18-2).

Acute pulmonary histoplasmosis is localized, mild, and self-limited and, with few exceptions, does not require therapy. In patients who have symptoms for more than 1 month, antifungal therapy may be helpful. Patients with mild-to-moderate acute pulmonary histoplasmosis who are symptomatic for more than 1 month may benefit from itraconazole for 6-12 weeks (Table 18-3). In patients with severe pulmonary histoplasmosis, a lipid formulation of amphotericin B for 1-2 weeks, followed by itraconazole

400 mg/d for a total of 12 weeks, is recommended. Itraconazole blood levels should be monitored after patient has received the antifungal for at least 2 weeks. Because patients with diffuse involvement may develop respiratory insufficiency caused by an inflammatory response during therapy, some experts add adjunctive corticosteroids for 2 to 3 weeks to diminish the inflammatory response. Clinical trials have not been able to demonstrate any significant difference in morbidity and mortality.

Patients with chronic cavitary pulmonary histoplasmosis merit treatment with itraconazole 200-400 mg/d for at least 12 months. Pericarditis associated with histoplasmosis should be treated with NSAIDS if the symptoms are mild and with itraconazole 200-400 mg/d for 6-12 weeks along with prednisone 0.5-1.0 mg/kg/d for the first 2 weeks. The antifungal is provided to reduce the incidence of possible dissemination during steroid therapy. Treatment for mediastinal lymphadenitis is generally unnecessary. However, if symptoms are severe, itraconazole 200-400 mg/d should be used if therapy with corticosteroids is warranted. Patients with either mediastinal granulomas or mediastinal fibrosis generally do not require antifungal therapy. If patients are symptomatic, itraconazole 200-400 mg/d should be used for 6-12 weeks. Surgery should be avoided in patients with mediastinal fibrosis, but these patients may benefit from vascular stenting if vascular obstruction is present. On the contrary, patients with mediastinal granulomas may require surgery to relieve the obstruction. Therapy with either antifungal should be used for 12 to 24 months (Table 18-3).

Therapy for disseminated disease is always required because the mortality of untreated infection ranges from 83% to 93%, whereas the mortality rate with therapy is between 7% and 23%. Liposomal amphotericin B (AmBisome®) 3 mg/kg/d or amphotericin B lipid complex (Abelcet®) 5.0 mg/kg/d for 1-2 weeks, followed by itraconazole 200-400 mg/d for at last 12 months, is the treat-

Table 18-3: Classification and Treatment of Histoplasmosis

Infection	Treatment
Acute Pulmonary Infection	
Mild	Symptoms <4 weeks: None Symptoms >4 weeks: Itraconazole 200-400 mg/d for 6-12 weeks;
Moderate–severe	Lipid amphotericin B 3-5 mg/kg/d or amphotericin deoxycholate 0.7-1.0 mg/kg/d x 1-2 weeks, de-escalate to itraconazole 400 mg/d x 12 weeks; methylprednisolone 0.5-1 mg/kg/d x 7-14 days;
Chronic cavitary pulmonary infection	Itraconazole 200-400 mg/d x 12 months
Pericarditis	
Mild	NSAIDS;
Moderate-severe	Itraconazole 200-400 mg/d x 6-12 weeks and prednisone 0.5-1 mg/kg/d x 1-2 weeks
Rheumatologic histoplasmosis	NSAIDS

NSAIDs=nonsteroidal anti-inflammatory drugs

ment of choice for fulminant disease. Patients with mild to moderate disseminated histoplasmosis may be treated with oral itraconazole 400 mg/d for at least 12 months. In patients with AIDS, because relapse is so predictable and occurs in more than 90% of cases, maintenance therapy

Infection	Treatment
Mediastinal lymphadenitis	Mild symptoms: None Itraconazole 200-400 mg/d and prednisone 0.5-1 mg/kg/d x 1-2 weeks
Mediastinal granuloma	Asymptomatic: None Symptoms: Itraconazole 200-400 mg/d x 6-12 weeks
Progressive disseminated histoplasmosis	
Mild	Itraconazole 200-400 mg/d x 12 months
Moderate-severe	Lipid amphotericin B 3-5 mg/kg/d or amphotericin B deoxycholate 0.7-1.0 mg/kg/d x 1-2 weeks, de-escalate to itraconazole 400 mg/d x 12 months.
CNS histoplasmosis	Lipid amphotericin B 5 mg/kg/d x 4-6 weeks, de-escalate to itraconazole 400-600 mg/d x 12 months.

with oral itraconazole 200 mg q.d. PO is recommended indefinitely. In these patients, serial antigen testing may prove beneficial in following the course of the disease. Fluconazole and ketoconazole should be used only if amphotericin B and itraconazole cannot be used.

CNS histoplasmosis includes meningitis, and lesions of the brain and/or spinal cord. All patients should be treated with liposomal amphotericin B 5 mg/kg/d for at least 4-6 weeks, followed by itraconazole 400-600 mg/d for a minimum of 12 months. Early and aggressive therapy should be undertaken because of the poor response rate and the high relapse rates.

Newer azole antifungals, such as voriconazole (Vfend®) and posaconazole (Noxafil®), and the echinocandins, such as caspofungin (Cancidas®), micafungin (Mycamine®), and anidulafungin (Eraxis™), have all demonstrated good in vitro activity and thus may prove to be useful alternatives in the future. Several in vivo animal trials with these agents have also demonstrated good results. Additionally, preliminary data from a multicenter clinical trial demonstrated that posaconazole has favorable activity against histoplasmosis unresponsive to other antifungal agents.

Suggested Readings

Deepe GS: Histoplasma capsulatum. In: Mandell GL, Bennett JF, Dolin R, eds. *Principles and Practice of Infectious Diseases.* 6th ed. New York, NY, Churchill Livingstone, 2005, pp 3012-3026.

Kaufmann CA: Histoplasmosis. In: Dismukes WE, Pappas PG, Sobel JD, eds. *Clinical Mycology.* 1st ed. New York, NY, Oxford University Press, 2003, pp 285-298.

Li RK, Ciblak MA, Nordoff N, et al: In vitro activities of voriconazole, itraconazole, and amphotericin B against Blastomyces dermatitidis, Coccidioides immitis, and Histoplasma capsulatum. *Antimicrob Agents Chemother* 2000;44:1734-1736.

Wheat J: Histoplasmosis: recognition and treatment. *Clin Infect Dis* 1994;19:S19-S27.

Wheat LJ, Connolly-Stringfield PA, Baker RL, et al: Disseminated histoplasmosis in the acquired immune deficiency syndrome: clinical findings, diagnosis and treatment, and review of the literature. *Medicine (Baltimore)* 1990;69:361-374.

Wheat LJ, Freifeld AG, Kleiman MB, et al: Clinical practice guidelines for the management of patients with histoplasmosis:

2007 update by the Infectious Diseases Society of America. *Clin Infect Dis* 2007;45:807-825.

Wheat J, Sarosi G, McKinsey D, et al: Practice guidelines for the management of patients with histoplasmosis. Infectious Diseases Society of America. *Clin Infect Dis* 2000;30:688-695.

Chapter 19

Coccidioidomycosis

Coccidioides immitis is a dimorphic fungus found predominantly in the southwestern United States and in northern Mexico. It is found in soil as clusters of filaments (hyphae) called mycelia, and as it matures, alternate cells along a hypha become barrel shaped. Hyphae with these structures are termed arthroconidia and are easily fragmented. These spores become airborne and can infect a new site in the soil. This cycle is known as the *saprophytic cycle*. In the host, the spores swell, become spherical, and develop a thick wall. These structures, known as spherules, reproduce by forming spherical internal spores called endospores. A single spherule may develop up to 800 endospores. The endospores are then released and form new spherules.

Epidemiology

Coccidioidomycosis is endemic to areas of North, Central, and South America and the United States. It is most common in the high Sonoran Desert and the southwestern United States. *Coccidioides immitis* is most prevalent along the San Joaquin Valley in California and in Arizona, New Mexico, Texas, and northern Mexico. In endemic areas, the annual risk of infection is approximately 3%. Miniepidemics have been described in association with archeological digs. Coccidioidomycosis is also endemic in some desert regions of the Western hemisphere, with seasonal distribution that follows drying out of the desert after rains. It is an occupational hazard among agricultural and construction

Table 19-1: Coccidioidomycosis Syndromes

- Pulmonary infection
  - Acute pulmonary infection
  - Chronic pulmonary infection (>3 mo)
- Disseminated infection
  - Cutaneous infection (~40%)
  - Musculoskeletal infection
  - Meningitis (~33%)

workers because disruption of soil releases spores. Factors that may predispose infected individuals to disseminated infection include pregnancy, age younger than 5 years or older than 50 years, and race, with Filipinos, Asians, and blacks being more affected than whites.

Pathogenesis

Infection is usually acquired by inhalation of aerosolized arthroconidia. Exposure to dust containing arthroconidia is therefore a main factor in determining exposure risk. Once inhaled, the fungus begins its dimorphic change in the lungs. Instead of reproducing by hyphal elongation, as in the soil, it develops into large spherules. The spherules undergo cleavage and form spherical internal spores, called endospores, which become new spherules. The identification of a mature endosporulating spherule in tissue is pathognomonic for *C immitis* infection. Hyphae can be found in pulmonary cavities along the interior margins in about 75% of cases. The primary tissue reaction is a granulomatous reaction.

Clinical Manifestations

There are three distinct clinical syndromes: acute pulmonary infection, chronic pulmonary infection, and disseminated infection (Table 19-1).

Acute Pulmonary Infection

The primary pulmonary infection is asymptomatic in approximately 60% of cases. In symptomatic cases, there is generally evidence of pulmonary infection, often with associated cutaneous lesions. The most common manifestations include a productive cough, pleuritic chest pain, malaise, fever, chills, night sweats, anorexia, weakness, arthralgia, and cutaneous lesions. Skin lesions include erythema nodosum, which occurs in about 2% to 10% of patients and primarily in females, and erythema multiforme, usually on the upper trunk and extremities.

About 1% of asymptomatic individuals with coccidioidomycosis develop symptomatic disease. This is more common in pregnant, immunocompromised, or dark-skinned patients, and it may result in miliary spread, with fatal consequences.

Most acute infections are transient and resolve spontaneously over a period of weeks. Chronic pulmonary lesions will persist in 10% of symptomatic patients. About 5% of patients develop residual lung disease with pulmonary nodules that may calcify. Other abnormalities that may be seen on chest radiograph include pulmonary infiltrates, hilar adenopathy, and thin-walled pulmonary cavities (Figure 19-1; see color plate insert). Most of these abnormalities also tend to resolve spontaneously without any sequelae.

Chronic Pulmonary Infection

Coccidioidomycosis that persists for more than 3 months is considered to be a chronic infection. In this setting, the acute pneumonic process does not resolve but instead progresses to a chronic pulmonary disease with cavities, nodules, or infiltrates (Figure 19-2; see color plate insert).

Nodules represent residual granulomatous reaction to a primary coccidioidal pneumonia. They tend to be solitary and 1 to 3 cm in diameter. Because most are caused by tissue reaction, they are generally asymptomatic and are often discovered during a routine chest radiograph. They are often confused with lung malignancy and are frequently resected. If the diagnosis of a coccidioidal nodule is made preoperatively, therapy is generally not required.

Cavitary coccidioidomycosis is usually caused by a secondary reaction to primary coccidioidal pneumonia. Cavitary lesions tend to be located in the periphery of the lungs and have thin walls. As with nodules, patients with these lesions are generally asymptomatic, and the cavity is discovered during routine chest radiograph. Cavities resolve spontaneously by 24 months in more than 50% of cases. Symptomatic patients may complain of productive cough with hemoptysis, pleuritic chest pain, malaise, and fever. Cavities may occasionally rupture into a bronchus or the pleural cavity and enlarge.

Coccidioidal infiltrates may progress and become chronic over time. These lesions frequently change character from infiltrates to cavities or nodules. Some infiltrates may continue to expand and involve multiple lobes and, occasionally, the opposite lung. Unlike patients with nodules or cavities, these patients are usually symptomatic and appear ill. Many complain of fever, malaise, fatigue, night sweats, anorexia, and weight loss. They may also have a productive cough with hemoptysis, pleuritic chest pain, and shortness of breath. As with other forms of chronic pneumonia, pulmonary tuberculosis and lung malignancies should be included in the differential diagnosis. In most cases, the manifestations do not resolve and the patient will require some form of therapy.

Disseminated Infection

Most cases of disseminated coccidioidomycosis are seen in immunocompromised patients, such as patients with diabetes, neutropenia, or HIV. In this setting, there is enhanced invasive potential with frequent reactivation and dissemination. Disseminated disease is also associated with rapid, diffuse, progressive pulmonary disease. Other groups at risk for higher rates of dissemination include pregnant women, especially those in their third trimester; Filipinos; and African Americans.

In areas where coccidioidomycosis is endemic, disseminated infection is often one of the most common AIDS-defining illnesses, and it can be life threatening without appropriate therapy. The most common risk factor in patients with AIDS appears to be the low CD4 cell count, generally <200 to 250 cells/μL. Once the CD4 cell count decreases to <200, the risk of disseminated infection increases 8 to 35 times.

Disseminated infection can occur in any organ, although it is most frequently seen in the lungs, skin, bones, joints, and meninges. In the lungs, the infection is characterized by diffuse reticulonodular or miliary infiltrates with associated respiratory failure.

Cutaneous disease is the most common form of disseminated disease. About 40% of patients with disseminated disease have cutaneous disease. The appearance of the lesions varies; large, verrucous lesions are common (Figure 19-3; see color plate insert), but papules, pustules, plaques, nodules, ulcers, and abscesses have been reported. The diagnosis can frequently be made by punch biopsy of the skin with fungal stains demonstrating the spherules.

Musculoskeletal infections often accompany disseminated disease. The infection can affect the muscles, tendons, and bones (about 60% unifocal). The most frequently affected areas include the vertebral column, pelvis, metacarpal bones, metatarsal bones, and lower extremities. The lesions are primarily lytic in nature. Joint involvement is unifocal more than 90% of the time, and the ankles and the knees are most commonly involved. Osteomyelitis is also common. The diagnosis is made by synovial biopsy that demonstrates a granulomatous reaction.

Meningitis is the most serious complication of disseminated infection and occurs in approximately one third of cases. It usually occurs within 3 to 6 months after primary infection and involves the basilar meninges. Mass lesions are uncommon. If left untreated, coccidioidal meningitis is fatal within 2 years. Manifestations include headaches, fever, weakness, confusion, sluggishness, seizures, nausea, and vomiting. Ataxia with focal neurologic deficits may also be seen. The cerebrospinal fluid usually demonstrates lymphocytic pleocytosis, hypoglycorrhachia, and an elevated protein level. Cultures may be negative. Complement-fixing antibodies to *C immitis* may be the only positive result.

Other sites of extrapulmonary coccidioidomycosis include the genitourinary tract, the prostate, the epididymis, and the tubo-ovarian and endometrial areas. Approximately 50% of genitourinary tract cases also involve the kidneys. The gastrointestinal tract is occasionally infected.

Obstetrical coccidioidomycosis is generally seen in endemic areas and is a leading cause of maternal mortality. The risk of disseminated infection is 40 to 100 times higher during pregnancy, and the mortality rate in pregnant patients is also much higher.

Diagnosis

Coccidioidomycosis is generally not difficult to diagnose, especially in endemic areas of infection. A mycologic diagnosis can be made with smears using potassium hydroxide or silver stains showing the spherules. Cerebrospinal fluid cultures are positive in about 33% of patients with meningitis. *Coccidioides immitis* grows well from clinical specimens in fungal media within 5 to 7 days.

Serologic examination may be the only indicator of disease in many infections. Two assays are commonly used to establish infection. The enzyme-linked immunosorbent assay for the mycelial-phase antigen coccidioidin is the most useful in detecting humoral antibodies. Serum IgG precipitins occur within 1 to 3 weeks after onset of infection in about 75% of patients and may disappear in approximately 4 months. Serum IgG appears in primary infection and may last in the serum for 6 to 8 months.

Table 19-2: Antifungals for Coccidioidomycosis

Drug	Route of Administration	Dose
Amphotericin B (Amphocin®, Fungizone®)	IV	1.0-1.5 mg/kg of body weight/d; decrease dose and frequency as improvement occurs
Lipid amphotericin B (AmBisome®, Abelcet®)	IV	3-5 mg/kg/d
Ketoconazole (Nizoral®)	Oral	400 mg/d
Itraconazole (Sporanox®)	Oral	200 mg twice a day with meals
Fluconazole (Diflucan®)	Oral	400-600 mg/d

Skin testing may also be used to identify infection. A reactive test indicates exposure at any time in the past and may not indicate active infection.

Management

The management of coccidioidomycosis is still controversial because many patients will have an acute, self-limited pulmonary infection that will resolve spontaneously without any form of therapy. However, most authorities

Comments

Systemic symptoms (eg, nausea, fever, myalgia) are common during infusions; side effects include nephrotoxicity, hypokalemia, and phlebitis; intravenous administration is inconvenient.

May have more gastrointestinal and other side effects than other azoles, and relapse rates may be higher than with itraconazole; liver toxicity occurs in rare cases; absorption requires acid and may be decreased if gastroenteropathy is present; drug interactions are less common than with itraconazole; tends to be less expensive than other azoles.

Interactions with several other drugs (eg, rifampin, phenytoin, cyclosporine); absorption may be a problem in some patients, as with ketoconazole.

Relapse rates appear to be higher than with itraconazole; drug interactions are less common than with itraconazole; the most expensive azole.

---

recommend antifungal treatment for all patients with symptomatic coccidioidomycosis.

Treatment may be difficult due to frequent relapses. In order to manage these infections, a standardized evaluation is used to assess overall severity (eg, symptoms, size, and number of lesions, serologic titers, cultures), in addition to factors that have been associated with an increased risk of complications. Antifungal management depends on the stage and site of the infection, especially with meningitis.

Table 19-3: Management of Coccidioidomycosis

Infection	Treatment
Pulmonary Infection	
Uncomplicated	Itraconazole 200 mg b.i.d., fluconazole 400 mg/d for 3-6 months.
Diffuse pneumonia	Lipid amphotericin B 3-5 mg/kg/d or amphotericin B deoxycholate 0.7-1.0 mg/kg/d or fluconazole 800 mg/d for 12 months.
Pulmonary nodule asymptomatic	No therapy recommended if lesion is completely resected.
Pulmonary cavity asymptomatic	No therapy recommended if lesion is completely resected.
Pulmonary cavity symptomatic	Itraconazole 200 mg b.i.d. or fluconazole 400 mg/d
Chronic Progressive Fibrocavitary Pneumonia	Itraconazole 200 mg b.i.d. or fluconazole 400 mg/d

Progression can be unpredictable, and remissions occur. Many infections may be refractory or may recur despite treatment with appropriate antifungals.

Available azoles such as fluconazole (Diflucan®) and itraconazole (Sporanox®) are the mainstays of antifungal therapy in most situations (Table 19-2). Most experts recommend antifungal therapy for 3 to 6 months, depending on the type and site of infection (Table 19-3). In patients with acute infection and no meningeal involvement, flu-

Infection	Treatment
Disseminated Infection	
Nonmeningeal	Itraconazole 400-800 mg/d or fluconazole 400-800 mg/d; lipid amphotericin B 3-5 mg/kg/d
Meningeal	Itraconazole 400-800 mg/d or fluconazole 400-800 mg/d; lipid amphotericin B 3-5 mg/kg/d. If poor response, consider the addition of intrathecal amphotericin B 0.1-1.5 mg per dose. Life-long therapy is recommended to prevent recurrences.

conazole 800 mg daily is the drug of choice. In patients with meningitis, therapy with fluconazole 800 mg daily is preferred. Patients who respond to this therapy will need to continue it for the rest of their life; recent studies indicate a high relapse rate in patients who discontinue therapy. If patients are refractory to fluconazole, then amphotericin B (Amphocin®, Fungizone®) may be administered intrathecally at a dose of 0.1 to 1.5 mg at daily to weekly intervals in addition to oral azole therapy. In most situations, the dose of amphotericin B is initiated at low levels and is increased gradually. Cerebrospinal fluid complement-fixing titers should be followed for evidence of resolution of the infection. Some patients may develop hydrocephalus as a complication of meningitis and may require a temporary or permanent ventricular shunt for decompression of the ventricles. Newer azoles voriconazole and posaconazole have also shown good activity against *C immitis* in vitro and in prelimary clinical trials.

Suggested Readings

Ampel NM: Coccidioidomycosis. In: Dismukes WE, Pappas PG, Sobel JD, eds. *Clinical Mycology.* 1st ed. New York, NY, Oxford University Press, 2003, pp 311-327.

Bouza E, Dreyer S, Hewitt WL, et al: Coccidioidal meningitis. An analysis of thirty-one cases and review of the literature. *Medicine (Baltimore)* 1981;60:139-172.

Dewsnup DH, Galgiani JN, Graybill JR, et al: Is it ever safe to stop azole therapy for *Coccidioides immitis* meningitis? *Ann Intern Med* 1996;124:305-310.

Galgiani J: Coccidioides species. In: Mandell GL, Bennett JF, Dolin R, eds. *Principles and Practice of Infectious Diseases.* 6th ed. New York, NY, Churchill Livingstone, 2005, pp 3040-3051.

Galgiani JN, Ampel NM, Blair JE, et al: Practice guideline for the treatment of coccidioidomycosis. Infectious Diseases Society of America. *Clin Infect Dis* 2005;41:1217-1223.

Galgiani JN, Catanzaro A, Cloud GA, et al: Comparison of oral fluconazole and itraconazole for progressive, nonmeningeal coccidioidomycosis. A randomized, double-blind trial. Mycoses Study Group. *Ann Intern Med* 2000;133:676-686.

Stevens DA: Coccidioidomycosis. *N Engl J Med* 1995;332:1077-1082.

Chapter **20**

Sporotrichosis

Epidemiology

Sporothrix schenckii is a dimorphic fungus that grows at room temperature on Sabouraud dextrose agar as a white mold, then turns brown to black with further incubation. It is isolated most often from soil, living plants, or plant debris.

Although *S schenckii* is found worldwide, most cases of sporotrichosis are reported from North and South America and Japan, and most infections occur as a result of direct contact with thorny plants such as roses and with sphagnum moss. Sporotrichosis is typically seen in miners, nursery workers, rose gardeners, Christmas tree farmers, and hay baling and masonry workers. Other, less common modes of infection include inhalation of conidia, leading to pulmonary sporotrichosis, and direct inoculation via bites or scratches from animals such as armadillos, cats, dogs, and birds. Additionally, several cases of sporotrichosis have occurred by direct inoculation of the organism in laboratory workers.

Clinical Manifestations

Sporotrichosis is an infection of cutaneous and lymphocutaneous tissues in 75% to 80% of cases. Although *S schenckii* is a true fungal pathogen producing disease in the immunocompetent host, the extent and the severity of infection vary with the host's immune status. The cutaneous form of infection is primarily seen in young adults, usually younger than 30 years. The extracutaneous forms of

Table 20-1: Forms of Sporotrichosis Infection

- Cutaneous and lymphocutaneous infections
- Extracutaneous infections
  - Osteoarticular infection
  - Pulmonary infection
  - Ocular infection
  - Disseminated infection

infection include disseminated, osteoarticular, meningeal, pulmonary, and genitourinary infections (Table 20-1). Patients with extracutaneous infection are generally older than 30 years, often without an obvious portal of entry but with a history of outdoor occupations. For unknown reasons, about one third of patients have a history of alcoholism. Other risk factors include diabetes mellitus, chronic lung disease, and HIV infection.

Cutaneous and Lymphocutaneous Sporotrichosis

Cutaneous or lymphocutaneous infection follows the direct introduction of organisms. Fungal growth is local, gradually extending proximally via the lymphatics and producing characteristic skin lesions. The incubation period is generally 7 to 14 days. There are two types of cutaneous syndromes: fixed, 'plaque-like' cutaneous sporotrichosis and lymphocutaneous sporotrichosis. Fixed cutaneous sporotrichosis is the least common form of infection, accounting for 10% to 20% of lesions. These lesions are generally confined to a single skin site and do not extend via the lymphatic channels. The lesions are plaque-like or verrucous and do not ulcerate (Figure 20-1; see color plate insert). Occasionally, the lesions resolve spontaneously.

In lymphocutaneous sporotrichosis, the lesion begins as a small, red, painless papule that enlarges slowly, becomes violaceous and nodular, intermittently produces a serosanguineous exudate, and is commonly followed by ulceration. The new lesions are characteristically nodular and tend to appear in the distribution of lymphatic channels proximal to the original site of infection. Lymphatic streaking between lesions is also common. The lesions are frequently painless or only mildly tender, and constitutional symptoms are generally absent. Occasionally, the infection may extend into deeper structures, producing tenosynovitis. This form of infection tends to be indolent and is frequently misdiagnosed for long periods.

Multifocal cutaneous sporotrichosis is uncommon but should be considered when the characteristic nodular lesions are seen beyond a single extremity and do not follow the lymphatic spread. This form of infection may be caused by hematogenous dissemination of the fungus.

These forms of sporotrichosis should be differentiated from infections caused by *Mycobacterium marinum*, nocardiosis, leishmaniasis, and tularemia, as well as other fungal infections such as blastomycosis, chromoblastomycosis, and paracoccidioidomycosis.

Extracutaneous Sporotrichosis

Most infections found outside the cutaneous and subcutaneous tissues are generally seen in immunocompromised patients.

Osteoarticular Sporotrichosis

These infections account for about 80% of all extracutaneous infections. The infection tends to involve the joints or bone, but it may also involve tendon sheaths and bursas in sites adjacent to cutaneous infections. It may follow contiguous spread from direct inoculation of the fungus.

Septic arthritis is more common than osteomyelitis and primarily involves the knee, elbow, wrist, ankle, and hand. The infection takes the form of an indolent arthritis that often is undiagnosed for a long time. Clinical manifestations include joint pain, decreased range of motion, effusion, edema, and minimal systemic or constitutional symptoms. Even with appropriate treatment, relapses are common, with poor functional outcome. The diagnosis is generally made with a positive culture of synovial fluid or synovial tissue.

Pulmonary Sporotrichosis

Pulmonary infection is uncommon and generally caused by inhalation of conidia into the respiratory tract. Most infections occur in older men with a history of alcoholism, smoking, or previously diagnosed chronic lung disease. Manifestations include productive cough, occasional hemoptysis, dyspnea, anorexia, weight loss, fatigue, and low-grade fever. The chest radiograph is often abnormal, demonstrating an indolent pneumonitis with or without cavitary lesions, primarily found in the upper lobes. The differential diagnosis should include tuberculosis, sarcoidosis, and other fungal infections such as histoplasmosis, blastomycosis, and coccidioidomycosis. If left untreated, the infection has a gradual and progressive course.

Ocular Sporotrichosis

Ocular infection is usually caused by traumatic inoculation of the eye. It primarily affects the conjunctiva, lids, lacrimal apparatus, and cornea. About 15% of cases will involve the orbits.

Disseminated Sporotrichosis

Disseminated infection generally presents with extensive lymphocutaneous lesions and occasional infection of visceral organs. Despite the increase in immunocompromised hosts, disseminated sporotrichosis remains rare.

However, when it does occur, it is generally associated with some degree of immunosuppression such as alcoholism, chemotherapy, and HIV infection. Most patients present with constitutional symptoms such as fever, chills, anorexia, malaise, and frequent atypical punched-out skin lesions. Although rare, meningitis may also develop with disseminated infection. These patients may present with indolent and persistent headaches, seizures, or alterations in mental status. Typically, meningitis caused by *S schenckii* is a difficult diagnosis to establish because cerebrospinal fluid (CSF) cultures are often negative. Examination of CSF shows an increase in white cells, with a lymphocytic predominance; a decrease in glucose; and an increase in protein. This form of meningitis is typically considered chronic, and it may take several lumbar punctures with analysis of large amounts of CSF to establish the diagnosis. Magnetic resonance imaging or computed tomography scans may show enhancing lesions in the brain tissue. In all cases of chronic meningitis, the differential diagnosis should include meningeal candidiasis, coccidioidomycosis, and tuberculosis.

Diagnosis

The diagnosis of sporotrichosis requires isolation of the fungus from affected tissues or material recovered from infected areas. Exudative material may be obtained by a swab of ulcerative lesions, skin biopsy, sputum, CSF, or blood.

On histopathology of infected tissue, granulomas are generally seen, with typical fungal cells that are confined to the dermis and surrounded by bodies that are positive on periodic acid-Schiff stain, forming the characteristic asteroid body of sporotrichosis. Special fungal stains are required to demonstrate *S schenckii* in specimens. However, because the tissues may have low levels of fungi, negative pathology specimens are not uncommon.

Table 20-2: Management of Sporotrichosis

Type of Disease	Preferred Treatment
Cutaneous, lymphocutaneous	Itraconazole (Sporanox®) 200 mg q.d. for 2-4 wk after lesions resolve
Pulmonary	Lipid amphotericin B 3.5 mg/kg/d for severe disease; itraconazole 200 mg b.i.d. for mild-to-moderate disease
Osteoarticular	Itraconazole 200 mg b.i.d. for 12 mo
Meningeal	Lipid amphotericin B 5 mg/kg/d x 4-6 wk
Disseminated	Lipid amphotericin B 3-5 mg/kg/d until clinical improvement
Disease in patients with AIDS	Amphotericin B deoxycholate 0.7-1.0 mg/kg/d until clinical improvement
	Lipid amphotericin B 3.5 mg/kg/d until clinical improvement

Several studies have evaluated enzyme-linked immunosorbent assays and CSF assays for the diagnosis of sporotrichosis. Although both of these assays have demonstrated good sensitivity and specificity, they are not readily available for routine clinical practice.

Alternative

Fluconazole (Diflucan®) 400-800 mg q.d.;
terbinafine (Lamisil®) 500 mg b.i.d.

Switch to itraconazole 200 mg b.i.d.
after the patient's condition has stabilized

Lipid amphotericin B 3.5 mg/kg/d or
amphotericin B deoxycholate 0.7-1.0 mg/kg/d

Switch to itraconazole after clinical response
to complete 12 months

Itraconazole 200 mg b.i.d. after amphotericin B
for suppression for a total of 12 months

Itraconazole 200 mg PO b.i.d. after amphotericin B
for suppression

Itraconazole 200 mg b.i.d. for suppression
for a total of 12 months

Itraconazole 200 mg b.i.d. for life-long suppression
or until immune reconstitution of HIV

Management

Unlike other forms of endemic infection, all forms of sporotrichosis require treatment. Because most cases are not life-threatening, oral azole antifungal therapy is the treatment of choice (Table 20-2). Saturated solution of potassium iodide (SSKI) was the standard of care for cutaneous and lymphocutaneous sporotrichosis for many years. Although effective, SSKI has a troublesome side effect profile, so the azole antifungals have replaced it as primary therapy. Itraconazole (Sporanox®) has become the drug of choice, with cure rates exceeding 90%. Other antifungal alternatives include the azoles, such as fluconazole (Diflucan®) and terbinafine (Lamisil®).

Pulmonary sporotrichosis responds poorly to any form of therapy. Occasionally, surgical excision or lobectomy, along with amphotericin B, must be considered.

Osteoarticular sporotrichosis responds slowly to antifungal therapy. Itraconazole 200 mg PO b.i.d. is the recommended regimen, which has an overall response rate of about 86%. Fluconazole is not as effective.

In disseminated sporotrichosis, lipid amphotericin B is the recommended antifungal of choice. However, once the patient responds to therapy and improves, he or she can be switched to itraconazole. HIV-positive patients, after responding favorably to initial therapy, should receive lifelong suppressive therapy with itraconazole because of their inherent immunosuppressed state.

Suggested Readings

al-Tawfiq JA, Wools KK: Disseminated sporotrichosis and *Sporothrix schenckii* fungemia as the initial presentation of human immunodeficiency virus infection. *Clin Infect Dis* 1998;26:1403-1406.

Kauffman CA, Bustamante B, Chapman SW, et al: Clinical practice guidelines for the management of sporotrichosis. 2007 update by the Infectious Diseases Society of America. *Clin Infect Dis* 2007; 45:1255-1265.

Kauffman CA, Pappas PG, McKinsey DS, et al: Treatment of lymphocutaneous and visceral sporotrichosis with fluconazole. *Clin Infect Dis* 1996;22:46-50.

Pappas PG: Sporotrichosis. In: Dismukes WE, Pappas PG, Sobel JD, eds. *Clincal Mycology.* 1st ed. New York, NY, Oxford University Press, 2003, pp 346-354.

Rex JH, Okhuysen PC: *Sporothrix schenckii.* In Mandell GL, Bennett JE, Dolin R, eds. *Principles and Practice of Infectious Diseases.* 6th ed. New York, NY, Churchill Livingstone, 2005, pp 2984-2988.

Sharkey-Mathis PK, Kauffman CA, Graybill JR, et al: Treatment of sporotrichosis with itraconazole. NIAID Mycoses Study Group. *Am J Med* 1993;95:279-285.

Chapter **21**

Paracoccidioidomycosis

Paracoccidioidomycosis (also known as South American blastomycosis) is a systemic fungal infection caused by the dimorphic fungus *Paracoccidioides brasiliensis*. *Paracoccidioides brasiliensis* is found exclusively in Latin America, especially in certain areas of Central and South America, from Mexico to Argentina, with Brazil at the center of the endemic region. For unknown reasons, it is not seen in Chile or in Caribbean countries. It appears to grow readily in areas with moderate temperatures, high humidity, and rich vegetation, although it has rarely been recovered from the soil in native regions.

Paracoccidioides brasiliensis exists as mycelia in nature and as yeast-like forms in tissue (37°C). The actual source of infection is unknown because the organism has been difficult to isolate from the environment. As with most endemic mycoses, the infection is acquired when conidia are inhaled into the respiratory tract, replicate, and produce the clinical syndromes associated with infection.

Paracoccidioidomycosis is unique among systemic mycoses because it is more common in men than women (15:1) and generally affects individuals older than 30 years. It is also common in agricultural workers and in those with a history of smoking cigarettes or drinking alcohol.

In addition, the infection has long periods of latency, which may last up to 30 years after primary infection.

Clinical Manifestations

Primary infection is frequently asymptomatic or subclinical, as with many of the endemic fungal infections. The organisms may remain latent within the lymph nodes of the thorax for years and reactivate during a period of immunosuppression. However, on occasion, the fungus can also disseminate outside the lungs to form ulcerative granulomas in other organs. The infection may be classified as acute, subacute (juvenile), or chronic and by the evolution and localization of lesions, which may be unifocal or multifocal in nature.

In adults, the most common presentation is pulmonary symptoms caused by the primary infection. Patients with pulmonary infection may complain of fatigue, malaise, weight loss, chest pain, and productive cough with occasional hemoptysis. They may also present with an ulcerative mucosal lesion that may affect any structure within the mouth, nose, and pharynx. The lesions begin as vesicles or papules that ulcerate, a condition known as 'moriform stomatitis.' The ulcerative lesions are painful and have a characteristic rolled border with a white exudative base and small hemorrhagic dots. The lesions are initially painless and then gradually spread, forming large vegetations. In severe cases, the lesions may advance and extend into deeper tissues, causing destruction of the uvula and hard palate. The tongue may also thicken and develop granulomatous nodules. Involvement of the lymph nodes in draining the affected area is also common, with frequent suppuration, drainage, and sinus tract formation. Other manifestations include dysphagia, odynophagia, and hoarseness.

As with other infections caused by dimorphic fungi, the infection may disseminate throughout the body. The predominant sites of extrapulmonary dissemination include the skin, mucous membranes, gastrointestinal tract, central nervous system, genitourinary tract, lymph nodes, adrenal glands, intestines, spleen, and liver.

In addition to the acute pulmonary infection, a chronic pulmonary infection may develop. Chronic infection is usually caused by reactivation of the primary focus of infection. In this setting, patients may have fever, weight loss, productive cough, anorexia, and malaise. These symptoms are accompanied by a variety of chest radiograph abnormalities, including solitary and multiple nodular lesions, cavitary lesions, and diffuse bilateral interstitial pulmonary infiltrates. On occasion, if duration of the infection is prolonged, fibrosis and bullae with parenchymal destruction may occur.

Diagnosis

Diagnosis is suspected clinically in endemic areas and confirmed by the isolation of the yeast form of the fungus from affected tissues. Frequently, a simple potassium hydroxide stain of sputum, pus, exudate, or biopsy material is the quickest way to establish the diagnosis. Isolation of the fungus should always be attempted. *Paracoccidioides brasiliensis* grows on Sabouraud dextrose agar, but it may take up to 7 to 10 days to reveal any significant growth.

Tissue biopsy is frequently diagnostic, and the histopathology of infected tissues may reveal a chronic granulomatous process.

Serology using the agar gel immunodiffusion assay is positive in approximately 95% of patients. It may be useful not only for diagnosis, but also for follow-up care of the infected patient.

Differential diagnosis should include other endemic mycoses, tuberculosis, and pulmonary malignancy.

Management

The overall outcome in patients in whom infection is diagnosed and treated early is good; however, therapy needs to be used for prolonged periods, usually 12 to 18 months.

This is the only fungal infection amenable to treatment with sulfonamides, which are used as acute therapy and as chronic suppressive therapy after amphotericin B (Amphocin®, Fungizone®).

In a recently completed clinical trial evaluating the efficacy of ketoconazole (Nizoral®), itraconazole (Sporanox®), and sulfadiazine for paracoccidioidomycosis in 42 patients, the investigators were unable to show any difference with any one regimen.

Overall, the azoles provide a significant advantage over sulfonamides. Ketoconazole, fluconazole (Diflucan®), and itraconazole have all demonstrated superiority in the management of paracoccidioidomycosis. Ketoconazole is effective at a dose of 200 to 400 mg/d for a prolonged period, usually 12 to 18 months. Current data, however, appear to favor the use of itraconazole at a dose of 200 mg/d as the treatment of choice, also for a prolonged period of time (3 to 12 months). Sulfadiazine or a long-acting sulfonamide may also be used as therapy, but the length of treatment should be at least 5 to 6 years to prevent relapses. Amphotericin B may also be used for severe cases, but it is not curative by itself and should be followed up with chronic suppressive therapy.

Suggested Readings:

Restrepo A: Paracoccidioides brasiliensis. In: Mandell GL, Bennet JE, Dolin R, eds. *Principles and Practice of Infectious Diseases*. 5th ed. New York, NY, Churchill Livingstone, 2005, pp 3062-3068.

Restrepo-Moreno A: Paracoccidioidomycosis. In: Dismukes WE, Pappas PG, Sobel JD, eds. *Clinical Mycology*. 1st ed. New York, NY, Oxford University Press, 2003, pp 328-345.

Shikanai-Yasuda MA, Benard G, Higaki Y, et al: Randomized trial with itraconazole, ketoconazole, and sulfadiazine in paracoccidioidomycosis. *Med Mycol* 2002;40:411-417.

Chapter 22

Miscellaneous Yeasts

Yeasts are ubiquitous in nature in plants, mammals, and insects. Accordingly, humans are continually exposed to many genera of yeast. Depending on the interaction between host mucosal defense mechanisms and fungal virulence factors, yeast colonization may be transient or persistent, systemic or local.

Yeast organisms usually have low virulence and often require a significant alteration or reduction in host defenses to successfully invade human tissue. Because the population of immunocompromised patients has recently increased, the incidence of yeast infections and the organisms causing them continues to grow (Table 22-1).

Protothecosis

Protothecosis is caused by a genus of ubiquitous, aerobic, unicellular achlorophyllic algae that exist as fungus-like saprophytes. There are three species: *Prototheca wickerhamii* (most common), *Prototheca zopfii*, and *Prototheca stagnora.*

Risk factors include hematologic malignancy (neutropenia), solid organ transplants, steroids, and diabetes. Occasionally, organisms may infect a normal host.

The route of infection is either cutaneous via traumatic inoculation or through the gastrointestinal (GI) tract. Several syndromes are associated with protothecosis.

Table 22-1: Miscellaneous Yeasts

- *Prototheca* spp
  - *P wickerhamii*
  - *P zopfii*
  - *P stagnora*
- *Malassezia furfur (Pityrosporum orbiculare)*
- *Trichosporon asahii (beigelii)*
- *Blastoschizomyces capitatus*
- *Rhodotorula* spp
  - *R mucilaginosa (rubra)*
  - *R glutinis*
- *Saccharomyces cerevisiae*

Microbiologic identification is the only way to identify *Prototheca* species. Morphologic identification may be made by using saline wet mounts. *Prototheca* species grow readily on Sabouraud dextrose agar and are easily identified using standard carbohydrate fermentation and assimilation profiles. It is often necessary to obtain a tissue biopsy to identify the organism in tissue.

Therapy, although controversial, includes surgical resection and excision of lesions along with the administration of amphotericin B (Amphocin®, Fungizone®). Although clinical trials have not been conducted, this form of therapy has been used successfully. Good results have also been seen with ketoconazole (Nizoral®), itraconazole (Sporanox®), and fluconazole (Diflucan®), especially in cutaneous infections. In patients with peritonitis due to continuous ambulatory peritoneal dialysis, the catheter should be removed and systemic antifungal therapy initiated.

Malassezia Infection

Malassezia furfur (*Pityrosporum orbiculare*, *Pityrosporum ovale*) is a common yeast frequently found on normal human skin. It causes superficial skin infections such as tinea (pityriasis) versicolor, dermatophytosis, and folliculitis; it occasionally causes fungemia and disseminated infection in the immunocompromised host.

Pathogens

Malassezia furfur is a dimorphic, lipophilic yeast that cannot synthesize medium- or long-chain fatty acids and has strict in vitro requirements for exogenous fatty acids of the C12 and C14 series. It exists primarily in the yeast form but may form superficial filamentous structures on the skin. Because of its nutritional requirements, *M furfur* is often not isolated from clinical specimens in the microbiology laboratory unless its presence is suspected and special preparations are made. *Malassezia pachydermatis* is generally associated with infections in dogs, in which it produces otitis externa. Both organisms produce clusters of oval to round thick-walled yeast cells, with unipolar buds that form repeatedly from the same pole of the parent cell. This gives rise to the characteristic 'collarette' at the bud site. Media such as Sabouraud dextrose agar require the addition of supplements such as olive oil in order to permit growth of *M furfur*. *Malassezia pachydermatis* does not require exogenous lipids for growth and can be recovered on standard fungal media.

In vitro susceptibility studies of *M furfur* strains report that most isolates are susceptible to amphotericin B, ketoconazole, miconazole (Micatin®, Monistat®), and fluconazole. However, most isolates are intrinsically resistant to flucytosine (Ancobon®).

Epidemiology

Malassezia furfur frequently colonizes the scalp, shoulders, chest, and back of normal hosts. The distribution of

Table 22-2: Risk Factors Associated With *Malassezia* Infections

- Prematurity
- Longer duration of hospitalization
- Use of occlusive dressings
- Administration of antibiotics
- Use of central venous catheters
- Use of intravenous lipids

colonization correlates with oily areas of the skin because the organisms require exogenous fatty acids, which they obtain from sebum. The highest incidence of colonization has been found in teenagers, with rates >90%.

Isolation of *M furfur* from newborns is reported to be <10% in nonintensive care settings but more than 80% in neonatal intensive care units. The reason may be that adult personnel routinely handle sick infants.

Although the epidemiology of disseminated infection has not been well studied, several risk factors are often associated with deep-seated infection by *M furfur* (Table 22-2).

Clinical Manifestations

Malassezia organisms produce superficial skin infections such as tinea (pityriasis) versicolor or a distinctive folliculitis and, occasionally, a deep-seated or hematogenous infection. The first reported case of systemic infection was described in 1981 in a premature neonate who developed vasculitis while on lipid therapy. Since then, there have been numerous reports describing disseminated infection.

The manifestations of disseminated or deep-seated infection vary from subclinical and mild symptoms, such as fever, to sepsis with multiorgan dysfunction. Most of these infections occur in premature infants, but they can occur in immunocompromised adults. The most commonly reported signs and symptoms of systemic infection include fever, bradycardia and respiratory distress (>50%), apnea (37%), hepatosplenomegaly (25%), and lethargy (12%). Laboratory findings include leukocytosis, thrombocytopenia, and bilateral pulmonary infiltrates (>50%).

Diagnosis

The diagnosis of disseminated infection can be made by gram stain of the buffy coat of blood. The budding yeast cells may be observed using specific fungal stains such as Giemsa, periodic acid-Schiff, or Calcofluor. Blood cultures will usually be negative, unless the infection is suspected and the laboratory adds sterile olive oil to the media. The recovery of the organisms may be enhanced by using lysis centrifugation. Blood culture tubes support the growth of the yeast.

Treatment

Management of *M furfur* fungemia and disseminated infection is controversial. Most authorities recommend prompt removal of the central venous catheter and discontinuation of intravenous lipids. In most cases without deep-seated infections, removal of the central venous catheter and discontinuation of lipids are all that is needed to clear the infection. This approach accomplishes two objectives: it eradicates the nidus of infection and removes the nutritional requirements of the organism. If fungemia persists or there is evidence of deep-seated infection, it is prudent to initiate antifungal therapy. Fortunately, *Malassezia* species are susceptible to azoles and polyenes. Although randomized clinical trials have not been undertaken, in most situations, fluconazole 400 mg/d or amphotericin B 0.7 mg/kg/d intravenously (IV) should be sufficient to eradicate the infection.

Trichosporonosis

Infections caused by organisms of the genus *Trichosporon* may be classified as superficial or deep. Superficial infection of the hair shafts is generally caused by *Trichosporon asahii* (*Trichosporon beigelii*) and is commonly known as white piedra because of its characteristic soft, white nodules. Deep-seated or disseminated infections have been recognized in the compromised host with increasing frequency over the past decade and are life threatening.

Trichosporon asahii was first described in 1865 by Beigel, who identified it as the causative agent of hair infection. The first reported case of disseminated infection appears to be a 39-year-old woman with adenocarcinoma of the lung who developed a brain abscess.

Pathogen

The genus *Trichosporon* was described by Behrend and has two species, *T asahii* (formerly *T beigelii, Trichosporon cutaneum*) and *Trichosporon capitatum. Trichosporon capitatum* is now called *Geotrichum capitatum* or *Blastoschizomyces capitatus*.

Trichosporon species are characterized by true hyphae, pseudohyphae, arthroconidia, and blastoconidia and are commonly found in soil and on animals and human skin. *Trichosporon asahii* grows readily on Sabouraud dextrose agar as rapidly growing, smooth, shiny gray to cream-colored colonies with cerebriform radiating furrows that become dry and membranous with age. It is readily identified using commercially available carbohydrate assimilation assays.

Epidemiology

Trichosporon asahii is generally found in the soil but can also be recovered from the air, rivers, lakes, sewage, and bird droppings. It rarely colonizes the inanimate environment but may colonize the mucosal surfaces of the oropharynx, the lower GI tract, and the skin in about 4% of humans.

Table 22-3: Risk Factors Associated With Trichosporonosis

- Underlying neoplastic disease
- Solid organ transplantation
- Neutropenia
- Use of broad-spectrum antibiotics
- Use of corticosteroids
- Bone marrow transplant

More than 100 cases of disseminated infection with *T asahii* have been documented. The major risk factors are included in Table 22-3. In most cases, the portal of entry appears to be the respiratory tract, the GI tract, or central venous catheters or percutaneous vascular devices.

Clinical Manifestations

Trichosporonosis can be classified into superficial infections, such as white piedra (hair shaft), onychomycosis, and otomycosis, and invasive infections. Invasive infection can be classified into localized deep-tissue infection and disseminated (hematogenous) infection. Deep-tissue infection results from the invasion of *Trichosporon* organisms into deep, nonmucosal tissues. The infection may involve a single organ or multiple organs. The most frequently affected organ is the lung, representing approximately 33% of localized deep-tissue infections. Other organs involved include the peritoneum, heart valves, eyes, brain, liver and spleen, stomach, kidneys, uterine tissue, gallbladder, and central nervous system (chronic fungal meningitis).

The clinical spectrum of disseminated infection resembles systemic candidiasis and includes fungemia associated with organ infection. Disseminated infections may be acute or chronic. Acute disseminated trichosporonosis often has a sudden onset and progresses rapidly, primarily in patients who are persistently neutropenic with fungemia characterized by persistent fever despite broad-spectrum antibacterial agents. Patients frequently develop cutaneous lesions (~33%), pulmonary infiltrates (30% to 60%), and hypotension with renal and ocular involvement.

The metastatic cutaneous lesions begin as an erythematous rash with raised papules on the trunk and the extremities. As the infection progresses, the rash evolves into macronodular lesions, followed by central necrosis of the nodules and, rarely, hemorrhagic bullae. Pulmonary infiltrates frequently accompany the disseminated infection and may be a lobar consolidation, bronchopneumonia, or a reticulonodular pattern.

Renal involvement in disseminated infection is common, occurring in >75% of cases. Renal disease may manifest as proteinuria, hematuria, red blood cell casts, acute renal failure, and glomerulonephritis. Urine cultures are frequently positive for *Trichosporon* organisms and should suggest disseminated disease in a neutropenic patient.

Chorioretinitis is seen in disseminated disease and may be a cause of decreased or complete loss of vision from retinal vein occlusion and retinal detachment. However, unlike candidal endophthalmitis, *Trichosporon* organisms infect uveal tissues, including the iris, and spare the vitreous.

During disseminated trichosporonosis, virtually any tissue in the body may become infected. Organs that have been documented to be involved include the liver, spleen, GI tract, lymph nodes, myocardium, bone marrow, pleura, brain, adrenal gland, thyroid gland, and skeletal muscle.

In chronic disseminated trichosporonosis, symptoms may be present for several weeks to months and include persistent fever despite broad-spectrum antimicrobials. The infection is similar to chronic disseminated (hepatosplenic) candidiasis. It tends to be a chronic infection of the liver, spleen, and other tissues after recovery from neutropenia. Laboratory studies frequently reveal elevated alkaline phosphatase. Imaging the abdomen with a computed tomography scan or magnetic resonance imaging reveals hepatic or splenic lesions compatible with abscesses. If lesions are demonstrated, a biopsy is needed to confirm the diagnosis.

Diagnosis

The diagnosis is made with a biopsy of the skin or involved organs that demonstrates the characteristic morphology of *Trichosporon* species. Blood cultures may be useful in diagnosing disseminated infection and deep-tissue infection. *Trichosporon* organisms will grow readily in blood culture and on fungal-specific media such as Sabouraud dextrose agar. The presence of *Trichosporon* organisms in the urine of a high-risk patient should increase the suspicion of disseminated infection.

Although there are no standardized serologic assays for *Trichosporon* species, the serum latex agglutination test for *Cryptococcus neoformans* may be positive.

Management

Trichosporonosis has a mortality rate of 60% to 70%. The underlying disease, persistent neutropenia, and concurrent infections contribute to overall mortality. Optimal therapy has not been established. Until recently, however, most patients received amphotericin B, occasionally in combination with flucytosine. Several investigators have reported amphotericin B resistant isolates of *T asahii*.

The initial step in the management of disseminated trichosporonosis should be to decrease or reverse immunosuppression.

Several new antifungal options are available. In vitro and animal models suggest that azoles and not polyenes are more effective in the eradication of *Trichosporon* species. In vitro susceptibility studies of *T asahii* reveal excellent activity with fluconazole and itraconazole. Although there are no established breakpoints to define resistance, most strains demonstrate relatively high minimum inhibitory concentrations (MICs) to amphotericin B.

Suggested therapy includes fluconazole 400 to 800 mg/d or itraconazole 400 to 600 mg/d for the treatment of disseminated trichosporonosis.

A second approach, especially in the non-neutropenic patient, is to use amphotericin B at 1.0 to 1.5 mg/kg/d. However, at these dosages, amphotericin B is fungistatic, not fungicidal. In a recent study in a murine model of disseminated trichosporonosis, the authors demonstrated that several antimicrobial combinations were superior to single-agent therapy using fluconazole or amphotericin B. The combination of fluconazole, amphotericin B, and levofloxacin (Levaquin®) appeared to be the most effective regimen in reducing fungal burdens in kidneys and improving survival in the murine model.

Among the newer triazoles, voriconazole (Vfend®), posaconazole (Noxafil®), and ravuconazole have demonstrated in vitro activity. All three agents were recently evaluated and demonstrated excellent in vitro activity against most isolates of *T asahii*. In a patient with disseminated infection, it may be clinically useful to determine in vitro susceptibilities as an adjunct in management, especially because recent case reports describe multidrug-resistant *T asahii* infections.

Blastoschizomyces capitatus

Infections with *B capitatus* (*T capitatum*), although not as common as those with *T asahii*, have been recognized in the immunocompromised host over the last 20 to 35 years. Most cases appear to be similar to disseminated candidiasis or disseminated *T asahii* infection. The isolates are difficult to differentiate from *Geotrichum candidum* and *T asahii*.

Blastoschizomyces capitatus is found in wood and poultry but has also been recovered from sputum and normal intact skin. Geographically, *B capitatus* infections occur more commonly in Europe, while *T asahii* infections occur in

North America. In most cases, the major risk factors include neutropenia and underlying hematologic malignancies.

The portal of entry is unknown but is suspected to be the respiratory tract, GI tract, and central venous catheters.

Clinical Manifestations

The infection may involve a single organ or multiple organs and may be associated with fungemia. The most frequently affected organs are the lungs, liver, skin, and central nervous system. Other organs involved include the spleen, epididymis, kidney, GI tract, vertebral bodies, and vertebral disk. Prosthetic heart valves may also be involved.

The clinical spectrum of disseminated infection is similar to that of systemic candidiasis and includes fungemia with or without organ infection. Generally, the manifestations begin with fever unresponsive to antimicrobials in a neutropenic patient. In the largest series from Italy, many patients presented with pulmonary disease characterized by cavitary lung lesions and focal hepatosplenic lesions. Skin lesions similar to those found in systemic candidiasis were also seen. Other, less commonly described infections include prosthetic valve endocarditis, urinary tract infection, vertebral osteomyelitis with diskitis of the lumbar spine, cerebritis, and brain abscess.

Diagnosis is made from positive blood cultures or from biopsy of the skin or affected organs. In a series from Italy, blood cultures were positive in 20 of 22 cases. *Blastoschizomyces capitatus* grows easily in blood culture bottles and on fungal media such as Sabouraud dextrose agar. Skin lesions are common but are generally negative on fungal stains and cultures.

Management

Infections with *B capitatus* have mortality rates between 60% and 70%. However, underlying disease, persistent neutropenia, and concurrent infections significantly contribute to overall mortality. Optimal therapy has not been established. Until recently, however, most patients received amphotericin B. In vitro susceptibility studies indicate that the organism seems to be susceptible to amphotericin B and itraconazole but less susceptible to azoles such as fluconazole and ketoconazole. Most isolates are resistant to flucytosine.

The initial step in the management of disseminated infection should be to decrease or reverse the immunocompromised state. Because most isolates are susceptible to amphotericin B, the recommendation is to use amphotericin B at a dose of 1.0 to 1.5 mg/kg/d. The newer azoles, voriconazole and posaconazole, also demonstrate good in vitro activity and may be suitable alternatives in the future.

Rhodotorulosis

Rhodotorulosis results from infection with *Rhodotorula* species. Although these yeasts are recovered worldwide from a variety of sources, infection is generally only seen in the immunocompromised host.

Rhodotorula rubra (*Rhodotorula mucilaginosa*) is the species most frequently associated with human infection. The other, less commonly isolated species include *Rhodotorula glutinis, Rhodotorula pilimanae, Rhodotorula pallida, Rhodotorula aurantiaca,* and *Rhodotorula minuta* (syn. *Rhodotorula marina*). Most *Rhodotorula* species produce red-to-orange colonies because of the presence of carotenoid pigments. The yeast readily grows on almost all types of culture media. In vitro susceptibility studies reveal that *Rhodotorula* species are susceptible to amphotericin B and are less susceptible to all azoles. However, posaconazole has shown in vitro activity against some *Rhodotorula* species. *Rhodotorula* species are also susceptible to flucytosine.

Epidemiology

Rhodotorula species are commonly recovered from seawater, plants, air, and food (cheese and milk products, fruit juices) and are occasionally recovered from humans. They are also recovered as an airborne laboratory contaminant. In addition, *Rhodotorula* organisms have been recovered from shower curtains, bathtub-wall junctions, and toothbrushes. In humans, *Rhodotorula* species have been recovered from the skin, nails, respiratory tract, urinary tract, GI tract, and blood stream.

Clinical Manifestations

Clinical signs and symptoms of the infection are nonspecific and vary from subtle and mild to severe, including septic shock. *Rhodotorula* species have been incriminated in a wide spectrum of infections, including blood stream infections, endocarditis, peritonitis, meningitis, and disseminated disease.

Rhodotorula fungemia is the most common form of infection. In most cases, it is associated with intravascular catheters in patients receiving either chemotherapy or long-term antimicrobials. Fever is the most frequent manifestation associated with fungemia.

Other forms of infection include endocarditis, central nervous system infections, and peritonitis. Three cases of *R rubra* peritonitis have been described in patients undergoing continuous ambulatory peritoneal dialysis. Environmental cultures revealed a possible common-source outbreak.

In most proven infections, *Rhodotorula* organisms are recovered from a sterile site of infection. In these cases, the decision to attribute a causal role to *Rhodotorula* is relatively simple, and the patient should be treated appropriately for an invasive fungal infection. However, this is not the case when the organism is recovered from body sites that may normally harbor *Rhodotorula* species, especially in the absence of signs or symptoms of infection. In this setting, it is necessary to establish true infection instead of colonization. *Rhodotorula* species readily grow in blood cultures and any media suitable for yeast, such as Sabouraud dextrose agar. Serologic diagnostic tests are not available.

Treatment

It is difficult to assess the role of antifungal therapy in patients with *Rhodotorula* infection. Optimal management of patients with indwelling catheters infected with *Rhodotorula* species has not been well defined. Several reports have documented clearance of fungemia and resolution of infection by removing the intravascular catheter in the absence of antifungal therapy. On the other hand, several reports suggest that antifungal treatment alone may suffice. Because *Rhodotorula* infections can be severe and life threatening, it is probably best to manage them aggressively by discontinuing the indwelling venous catheter if possible and using systemic antifungal therapy.

Saccharomyces Species

Saccharomyces is a genus of ascomycetous yeasts that are widespread in nature. It includes *Saccharomyces cerevisiae* (*Saccharomyces carlsbergensis*) and *Saccharomyces fragilis.* Some species are occasionally part of the normal flora of the GI and genitourinary tracts. *Saccharomyces cerevisiae*, also known as brewer's yeast or baker's yeast, has been reported to cause infection in humans. It is better known for its commercial uses: beer and wine production, health food supplementation, and DNA recombinant technology. Recently, it has been found to cause mucosal and disseminated infection in humans.

In most cases, the organisms are nonpathogenic because they have innate low virulence. In early experimental studies, subcutaneous inoculation with *S cerevisiae* was neither lethal nor invasive for normal and cortisone-treated mice. More recent studies have demonstrated that some clinical isolates of *S cerevisiae* in CD-1 mice can proliferate and resist clearance in vivo. Thus, these studies support *S cerevisiae* as a cause of clinical infection. In vitro susceptibility studies reveal that *S cerevisiae,* compared to *Candida albicans* isolates, is less susceptible to most antifungals, including azoles.

Epidemiology

Recovery of *Saccharomyces* species from human mucosal surfaces is rarely clinically significant, but isolation from sterile body sites has been described. *Saccharomyces* organisms have been recovered from the blood stream, lungs, peritoneal cavity, esophagus, urinary tract, and vagina.

Recent DNA typing studies evaluating the relation between clinical strains and commercial strains of *S cerevisiae* have demonstrated that commercial products may be a contributing factor in human colonization and infection.

The risk factors associated with *Saccharomyces* infections are similar to the risk factors associated with candidemia and systemic candidiasis, including central venous catheters, neutropenia, antimicrobial use, and GI tract surgery. There have also been several reports of *S cerevisiae* fungemia in HIV-positive patients. Possible portals of entry for invasive disease include the oropharynx, GI tract, and skin.

Clinical Manifestations

Clinical signs and symptoms of infection are nonspecific and vary from subtle and mild to severe. *Saccharomyces* species have been incriminated in blood stream infections, endocarditis, peritonitis, disseminated disease, pneumonia, and vaginitis.

Fungemia, the most common form of infection, is seen in the immunocompromised host and is associated with intravascular catheters, chemotherapy, and antimicrobial use. Manifestations are similar to those of systemic candidiasis and candidemia. Fever of unknown etiology is the most frequent symptom associated with fungemia, and in most cases, the patients have survived.

There have been several reported cases of respiratory tract infection. Most occur in patients with underlying hematologic malignancies. There have also been several cases of empyema. In one patient, empyema resulted from a complication during sclerotherapy for esophageal varices.

In several cases, *S cerevisiae* was recovered from the peritoneal fluid of symptomatic patients who underwent surgery for malignant neoplasms. The patients were cured with surgical drainage and antifungal therapy. There has been one reported case of cholecystitis in a patient with diabetes mellitus. The isolate was recovered from the gallbladder and from the stone inside the gallbladder.

There have been three documented cases of endocarditis, all associated with prosthetic valves. Two of these patients were intravenous heroin users. All three patients were apparently cured with antifungal therapy; in only one patient was the valve replaced.

Genitourinary tract infections are more common than invasive infections. Several cases of urinary tract infection and of fungus balls with *S cerevisiae* have been reported. Renal abscesses associated with fungemia have also been documented. Even more common is vaginitis caused by *S cerevisiae. Saccharomyces cerevisiae* has been reported in more than 25 women who suffered from refractory vaginitis.

Diagnosis

The patient with *S cerevisiae* infection should be treated for an invasive fungal infection. Diagnostic difficulty occurs when the organism is recovered from body sites that may be colonized by *Saccharomyces* organisms, especially in the absence of symptoms of infection. In this setting, it is necessary to establish true infection instead of colonization. *Saccharomyces cerevisiae* readily grows from blood culture bottles and on Sabouraud dextrose agar.

Treatment

As with many nonpathogenic yeast infections, it is difficult to assess the role of antifungal therapy in patients infected with *Saccharomyces* organisms. Optimal management of patients with prosthetic valve infections and infected indwelling catheters has not been established.

Several reports document clearance of fungemia and resolution of infection by removing the intravascular catheter without providing antifungal therapy. Most experts advocate removal of the indwelling catheter and use of antifungal agents. *Saccharomyces* species are susceptible to most antifungals, including amphotericin B, flucytosine, ketoconazole, clotrimazole (Lotrimin®), miconazole, terconazole (Terazol® 3, Terazol® 7), voriconazole, and posaconazole.

Suggested Reading

Hazen KC: New and emerging yeast pathogens. *Clin Microbiol Rev* 1995;8:462-478.

Hospenthal DR: Uncommon fungi. In: Mandell GL, Bennett JE, Dolin R, eds. *Principles and Practice of Infectious Diseases.* 6th ed. New York, NY, Churchill Livingston, 2005, pp 3068-3079.

Vazquez JA: Rhodotorula, Malassezia, Trichosporon, and other yeast-like fungi. In Dismukes WE, Pappas PG, Sobel JD, eds. *Clinical Mycology.* 1st ed. New York, NY, Oxford University Press, 2003, pp 206-217.

Chapter **23**

Chromoblastomycosis

Chromoblastomycosis is a gradually progressive and debilitating cutaneous and subcutaneous fungal infection caused by a group of dematiaceous fungi. The infection is found worldwide, but most cases occur in tropical and subtropical regions. The infection is caused by the traumatic implantation of one of the fungi into the skin or subcutaneous structures.

The main etiologic agents, from most common to least common, include *Fonsecaea pedrosoi*, *Cladosporium carrionii*, *Fonsecaea compacta*, *Phialophora verrucosa*, and *Rhinocladiella aquaspersa*. Most of these organisms are found in soil and planting materials.

The lesions tend to remain localized to the area of implantation, although hematogenous dissemination in the compromised host has been reported. There are five types of lesions described in the literature. The nodular lesions are elevated and soft. These dull-to-pink growths may be smooth, scaly, or verrucous. This type of lesion may progress to the tumorous type of lesion. The tumorous lesion tends to be larger and is frequently covered by dirty gray epidermal debris and crusting (Figure 23-1; see color plate insert). These lesions may also be lobulated or papillomatous. The verrucous lesions have the characteristics of warts and are commonly seen along the borders of the foot. The plaque lesions are flat and scaly, with a reddish to violaceous color. The cicatricial lesions enlarge by expansion with central scarring and healing.

The diagnosis can be made by either a 10% potassium hydroxide stain of crusted material, demonstrating dematiaceous, septate, branching hyphae, or by culture of purulent discharge or tissue. On histopathology, the skin lesions will characteristically show hyperkeratous hyperplasia and microabscesses in the epidermis. The dematiaceous hyphae and sclerotic bodies are found in the stratum corneum.

Treatment

The treatment of chromoblastomycosis is frequently difficult and unsatisfactory. The early stages of infection are treated with surgical excision, electrodesiccation, cryosurgery, or topical antifungals. In advanced cases, systemic antifungal therapy is required for prolonged periods of time. Itraconazole (Sporanox®) 200 to 400 mg/d or terbinafine (Lamisil®) 250 mg PO q.d. for prolonged periods of time has been successful. Clinical trials with fluconazole (Diflucan®) have been disappointing. The newer triazole, voriconazole (Vfend®), appears to have good in vitro activity and may need to be evaluated in clinical trials. Additionally, posaconazole has shown favorable activity in vitro, and in patients with chromoblastomycosis refractory to other therapies.

The most promising form of therapy appears to be the combination of antifungal agents plus surgical debridement or cryotherapy.

Suggested Reading

Baddley JW, Dismukes WE: Chromoblastomycosis. In: Dismukes WE, Pappas PG, Sobel JD, eds. *Clinical Mycology.* 1st ed. New York, NY, Oxford University Press, 2003, pp 399-404.

Hospenthal DR: Agents of Chromoblastomycosis. In: Mandell GL, Bennett JE, Dolin R, eds. *Principles and Practice of Infectious Diseases.* 6th ed. New York, NY, Churchill Livingstone, 2005, pp 2988-2991.

Rex JH, Stevens DA: Systemic antifungal agents. In: Mandell GL, Bennett JE, Dolin R, eds. *Principles and Practice of Infectious Diseases.* 6th ed. New York, NY, Churchill Livingstone, 2005, pp 502-513.

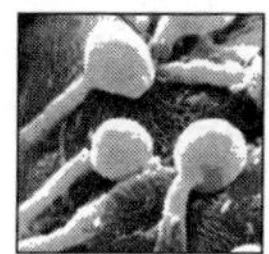

Index

B

C

D

E

F

G

H

I

J

K

L

M

N

O

P

Q

R

S

T

U

V

W

Y

Z

NOTES

NOTES

NOTES